THE MENOPAUSE UNICORN

CONQUER HORMONES, RECLAIM YOUR HEALTH, AND THRIVE LIKE A BADASS

KIM STEGEMAN

© **Copyright 2025 - All rights reserved.**

The content within this book may not be reproduced, duplicated or transmitted without direct written permission from the author or the publisher.

Under no circumstances will any blame or legal responsibility be held against the publisher, or author, for any damages, reparation, or monetary loss due to the information contained within this book. Either directly or indirectly. You are responsible for your own choices, actions, and results.

Legal Notice:

This book is copyright protected. This book is only for personal use. You cannot amend, distribute, sell, use, quote or paraphrase any part, of the content within this book, without the consent of the author or publisher.

Disclaimer Notice:

Please note the information contained within this document is for educational and entertainment purposes only. All effort has been expended to present accurate, up-to-date, and reliable, complete information. No warranties of any kind are declared or implied. Readers acknowledge that the author is not engaging in the rendering of legal, financial, medical or professional advice. The content within this book has been derived from various sources. Please consult a licensed professional before attempting any techniques outlined in this book.

By reading this document, the reader agrees that under no circumstances is the author responsible for any losses, direct or indirect, which are incurred as a result of the use of the information contained within this document, including, but not limited to, — errors, omissions, or inaccuracies.

CONTENTS

Introduction   7

1. UNDERSTANDING THE MENOPAUSAL TRANSITION   13
   1.1 Demystifying Menopause: A Biological Overview   14
   1.2 From Perimenopause to Postmenopause: Navigating the Phases   16
   1.3 Hormonal Havoc: Understanding Estrogen, Progesterone, and More   19
   1.4 The Emotional Landscape: Mood Swings and Mental Health   21
   1.5 Debunking Myths: Separating Fact from Fiction   25
   1.6 Societal Stigmas and Breaking the Silence   28
   1.7 The Power of Knowledge: Preparing for Your Journey   31

2. MASTERING EVERYDAY SYMPTOM RELIEF   34
   2.1 Hot Flash Hacks: Staying Cool Under Pressure   35
   2.2 Sleep Solutions: Overcoming Insomnia and Night Sweats   38
   2.3 Mood Balancing Act: Emotional Well-being and Stability   42
   2.4 Weight Wisdom: Tackling Menopausal Weight Gain   45
   2.5 Libido Liberation: Reigniting Intimacy and Connection   49
   2.6 Lesser-Known Symptoms: Identifying and Managing Surprises   52

3. NOURISHING YOUR BODY: NUTRITION AND LIFESTYLE   59
   3.1 Nutritional Needs: Feeding Your Changing Body   59
   3.2 Exercise Essentials: Staying Active and Strong   71
   3.3 Mindful Eating: Listening to Your Body's Signals   78

    3.4 Superfoods for Menopause: What to Add to
Your Diet   81
    3.5 Hydration and Health: The Importance of
Water   85
    3.6 Alcohol and Caffeine: Friends or Foes?   87

4. STARTING POINTS: NATURAL, ALTERNATIVE,
AND EMERGING THERAPIES   94
    4.1 Acupuncture and Acupressure: Eastern Relief
for Western Symptoms   95
    4.2 Herbal Remedies: An Evidence-Based
Approach   99
    4.3 Adaptogens: Focusing on Stress Management   102
    4.4 The Role of Supplements: Finding the Right
Boost   108
    4.5 New and Innovative Therapies: Expanding the
Treatment Landscape   111
    4.6 Wrapping Up: Building Your Toolkit, Layer by
Layer   115

5. HORMONE REPLACEMENT THERAPY: THE
GOLD STANDARD FOR MENOPAUSE CARE   119
    5.1 Intro to Hormone Replacement Therapy   120
    5.2 The Benefits and Risks (and the Truth About
that WHI Study)   121
    5.3 Systemic vs. Local HRT   123
    5.4 Bioidentical Hormones: What They Are—and
What They Aren't   123
    5.5 Natural vs Synthetic: Cutting Through the
Confusion   124
    5.6 FDA-Approved vs Compounded Bioidentical
Hormones   126
    5.7 My Experience with HRT   128
    5.8 The Bottom Line   129

6. BUILDING A SUPPORTIVE HEALTH TEAM   132
    6.1 Finding the Right Doctor: Advocacy and
Communication Tips   132
    6.2 The Menopause Coach: A Guide to
Professional Support   135
    6.3 Empowering Conversations: Speaking Up
About Symptoms   138
    6.4 Understanding Healthcare Options: Making
Informed Choices   140

6.5 Insurance Insights: Navigating Coverage and Costs   141
6.6 Building Your Support Network: Family, Friends, and Professionals   145

7. EMBRACING EMOTIONAL AND MENTAL WELLNESS   149
7.1 Your New Toolkit: Preparing for Your Emotional and Mental Journey   149
7.2 Mindfulness and Meditation for Menopause: Finding Your Inner Peace   150
7.3 Self-Care Strategies: Prioritizing Your Well-being   155
7.4 Creating a Menopause Journal: Tracking Your Journey   160
7.5 The Art of Letting Go: Embracing Change and Transformation   166

8. REVITALIZING RELATIONSHIPS AND INTIMACY   172
8.1 Love in the Time of Menopause: Nurturing Relationships   172
8.2 Honest Conversations: Talking About Menopause with Partners   176
8.3 Sexual Health: Addressing Changes and Enhancing Pleasure   179
8.4 Reconnecting with Yourself: Self-Exploration and Confidence   182
8.5 Navigating Family Dynamics: Sharing Your Experience   186
8.6 Empty Nest and Beyond: Redefining Your Role   189

9. THRIVING THROUGH PERSONAL GROWTH AND TRANSFORMATION   195
9.1 Embracing New Passions: Finding Joy in Reinvention   196
9.2 Setting New Goals: Crafting Your Menopause Vision   197
9.3 Building Resilience: Strengthening Your Inner Badass   200
9.4 Celebrating Your Journey: Milestones and Achievements   203

9.5 The Menopause Unicorn: Thriving Against
All Odds   205
9.6 Empowering the Next Generation: Sharing
Your Wisdom   208

Conclusion   213
References   217

INTRODUCTION

Fall 2022—I hit what felt like rock bottom. My body, once an ally, had turned against me. I was limping with plantar fasciitis, tipping the scale at 274 pounds, and dragging myself to the gym two or three times a week, hoping for a miracle. Instead, I was exhausted, irritable, and so far from feeling sexy that my poor husband probably felt like he needed a game plan every time he approached me. Would I be raging? Prickly? Weepy? Sore? Or was I just plain grouchy because I felt so awful in my own skin?

On top of that, I was leading the world's largest roller derby organization out of a global pandemic—an unbelievably stressful gig—and my tank was completely empty. My mental fortitude was hanging by a thread, my confidence was in the dumps, and my physical discomfort only made it all worse. This wasn't burnout—it was like my body and mind had formed a union and gone on strike. Something had to give.

Desperate for answers, I finally dragged myself to my doctor. What I got felt like advice straight out of the 1980s: "Have you considered a box food diet?" There were no labs, no hormone tests, and no questions about what I was really experiencing—

just processed meals and a pat on the back. I left feeling dismissed, unseen, and furious. That was the moment I realized I needed a new plan—and a new doctor.

I turned to my friend Emily Howell, a trainer at the Bay Club who'd been through her own hormonal chaos. She's now a certified menopause coach and Women's Coaching Specialist (WCS). Emily is the person I credit with putting me on this amazing path. She's an incredible trainer—I loved lifting with her. She leads by example, lifting heavy in her own workouts and staying laser-focused on fueling her body right. When I felt like a stranger in my own skin, she recommended Dr. Bourgeois, a naturopath. The catch? A three-month wait. So, I grabbed a journal and made a vision board for the life I wanted to build. That small act of intentionality—putting my goals on paper—felt like the first step toward reclaiming my body, mind, and confidence.

I've spent 20 years building a badass community of women and non-binary skaters, and now I'm channeling that same fire into helping you tackle menopause—with humor, honesty, and zero bullshit.

Fast forward 18 months to mid-2024. I've dropped weight (60+ lbs.), gained energy, and feel better than ever. People stop me and ask, "What's your secret?" My answer? "It's menopause—it's really working for me. I'm a Menopause Unicorn."

But how did I get here? That's what this book is about.

The Menopause Unicorn isn't just a playful metaphor. It's a symbol of thriving when the world tells you to settle. It's about rewriting the menopause narrative—trading dread for curiosity and fear for empowerment. It's about finding the magic in this transition and owning it like the badass you are.

Menopause is the beginning of a bold, new chapter. It's your chance to hit reset, rediscover who you are, and build the life you truly want. Whether you're reinventing yourself, exploring new passions, or simply learning how to feel good in your skin again, this book will walk alongside you every step of the way.

If you're a woman between 35 and 55, ready to tackle menopause with humor, resilience, and confidence, you're in the right place. Curious about HRT? Love the idea of natural remedies? Just need someone to remind you you're not alone? This book is for you.

This book is your roadmap for thriving—not just surviving—menopause. You'll learn how to manage symptoms, explore treatment options (from hormones to herbs), fuel your body, care for your emotional health, and reinvent yourself. Whether you're curious about natural remedies, passionate about strength training, or just trying to make sense of all the changes, you'll find the tools, encouragement, and stories you need to build a plan that works for you.

Here's are some elements of the book you'll love:

- **Managing Symptoms** – We'll tackle it all, from hot flashes to brain fog.
- **Exploring Treatments** – Whether you choose HRT, herbs, or mind-body practices like yoga and meditation, you'll have the tools to create a personalized plan.
- **Nutrition and Fitness** – Fuel your body and build strength to feel unstoppable.
- **Emotional Wellness** – Strategies for managing stress, mood swings, and relationships.
- **Family Dynamics** – Tips for navigating the chaos at home with humor and grace.

- **Sex, Confidence, and Reinvention** – Because menopause isn't just about survival; it's about thriving in every area of your life.

You'll also find encouragement to:

- Advocate for yourself with doctors.
- Build supportive communities.
- Celebrate the wins—big and small.
- Create a routine that works for you.

I wrote this book because I believe menopause doesn't have to be feared or dreaded. It can be a transformation, a superpower, and—yes—even magical.

So, let's dive in. Let's discard the shame, outdated advice, and the idea that you're "past your prime."

This is your time. Your reset. It's your moment to thrive like the badass you are and become your own Menopause Unicorn.

First up: understanding what the heck is actually going on with your body—because no, you're not imagining it. Chapter 1 cracks open the black box of menopause: the biology, the phases, the hormones, the emotional rollercoaster, and all the BS myths we've been spoon-fed since puberty. This is the chapter I wish someone had handed me five years ago and said, "Here. Read this. It's not you, it's your hormones. And there's a way through."

Are you ready? Let's do this.

1

UNDERSTANDING THE MENOPAUSAL TRANSITION

Before we start diving into treatments, supplements, or whether you should burn your underwire bras and start a new life in Bali, we need to start with the basics. Because here's the deal: you can't tackle something if you don't understand what is happening in your own body.

We're going to look under the hood and name what's going on —because knowledge isn't just power. It's *freedom*. Freedom from shame, confusion, and gaslighting from doctors who think you just need a new diet or a vacation.

If you're ready to finally understand what your body is doing— and why you sometimes want to cry, scream, or move to a yurt in the woods—you're in the right place. Let's start by demystifying menopause. Spoiler alert: it's not all doom and dryness.

1.1 DEMYSTIFYING MENOPAUSE: A BIOLOGICAL OVERVIEW

What comes to mind when you hear the word *menopause*? Hot flashes? Mood swings? Crying in a Costco parking lot and wondering if you're losing your mind?

Same. But the truth is, menopause isn't just about night sweats and forgetting why you walked into a room. It's about change—messy, powerful, sometimes infuriating change. But when you understand *what's* happening in your body, you get to take the wheel instead of riding shotgun on a runaway hormone train.

Menopause is a natural biological transition, not a disease or a failure. But most of us are left to stumble through it with half-baked advice, bad Google searches, and doctors who think "just wait it out" is an actual treatment plan.

Let's start with the facts.

Wait—What Is Menopause, Really?

Here's where things get confusing: **menopause** is technically just one moment in time—the day you've gone *12 full months* without a period. Everything *before* that? That's **perimenopause**, when your hormones start shifting, sputtering, and throwing you curveballs. Everything *after*? That's **postmenopause**, the new normal your body settles into.

But most people use "menopause" to describe the whole messy arc—from the first weird symptoms to well beyond the last tampon. So in this book, we'll use it both ways—clinically when it matters, casually when it makes more sense.

Estrogen and Progesterone: The Unsung Heroes

Before perimenopause kicks off, your ovaries are cranking out estrogen and progesterone on a predictable rhythm. These hormones do *way* more than regulate your period. They help stabilize your mood, protect your bones and heart, support brain function, influence sleep, and keep your vaginal tissue supple and healthy. (Yes, that's a thing.)

When those hormone levels start to decline—and fluctuate wildly on the way down—your body notices. Even if *you* don't realize what's happening yet.

The Symptoms Are Sneaky

The symptoms? Wildly diverse—and often surprising. Some are headline-grabbers (hot flashes, anyone?), but others creep in quietly: anxiety that hits out of nowhere, brain fog that messes with your memory, or new food sensitivities that make no sense. If your body suddenly feels unfamiliar, you're not alone— and we'll dig into the specifics in the next section.

These aren't random. They're part of a larger picture—and that picture starts to make sense once you understand the hormonal shifts behind it.

You're not imagining it. You're not overreacting. Your body is changing. And the more you understand it, the more empowered you'll be to respond instead of just endure.

Every Menopause Journey Is Different

Some people sail through with barely a symptom. Others feel like their body is staging a full-blown rebellion. Genetics, lifestyle, stress, and overall health all influence the ride.

So if your friend swears by herbal tea and breathing exercises, while you're sleeping on a frozen towel, both experiences are valid. Your journey is yours. No shame, no comparison, no one-size-fits-all timeline.

Menopause as a Catalyst

Yes, this transition can be brutal. But it can also be liberating. Menopause invites you—*forces* you, really—to slow down, tune in, and recalibrate. It can be the start of something powerful:

A fresh chapter. A permission slip. A middle finger to expectations you've outgrown.

Whether you're rebuilding your health, reclaiming your identity, or just trying to survive without punching someone in the produce aisle, this is your time.

1.2 FROM PERIMENOPAUSE TO POSTMENOPAUSE: NAVIGATING THE PHASES

Let's break this transition down. Menopause isn't one big hormonal "event"—it's a *process*. A long, often messy, and wildly personal one. Understanding the different phases can make the chaos feel a little less... chaotic.

Perimenopause: The Sh*t Gets Weird Phase

Perimenopause is the lead-up—the runway, if you will. It can start years before your periods stop entirely. Estrogen and progesterone start to fluctuate like a toddler with a light switch, and your body reacts in kind. As Dr. Kaley Bourgeois, Naturopathic Physician (ND) at Famework Integrative Medicine in Oregon, points out, key indicators of perimenopause include changes in sleep, energy levels, exercise endurance, memory issues (particularly word recall), emotional regulation, temperature sensitivity, joint pain, and weight fluctuations. Some of these changes come on gradually, which can lead both patients and doctors to overlook that this may be the start of perimenopause.

On top of that, your cycle might go MIA for a few months, then show up with a vengeance. One month it's light and breezy, the next it's a murder scene. You might feel foggy, anxious, ragey, or all three *in one afternoon*. Sex might feel different, your skin might change, your hair might get dry, and your favorite foods might suddenly betray you.

Basically, your body is remixing itself—and the playlist is unpredictable.

"Perimenopause is unpredictable. There's this idea that if you just see the right provider or do the right test, you'll have clarity—but we won't. We are all on our own ride," says Christina Cameli, CNM, owner of Menopause NW, a midwife and menopause practitioner.

Menopause: The Milestone Moment

This phase gets all the name recognition, but it's actually *just one day*—the 12-month mark with no period. You won't know you're there until you look back and say, "Oh. It's been a year."

By this point, many of the symptoms you've been riding through may start to ease. (Or not. Thanks, body!) You might feel a little more like yourself—or like a *new* version of yourself, one you're just getting to know.

Postmenopause: The Long Game

Once you've crossed the one-year threshold, welcome to postmenopause. This is your new hormonal baseline—and with it comes a new set of considerations.

Estrogen continues to decline, which can raise your risk of things like bone loss, heart disease, and shifts in cholesterol levels. This is the time to start thinking long-term: bone density, strength training, heart health, mental health. Not out of fear—but out of love for the future you.

What to Expect (Besides the Unexpected)

Everyone's experience is different, but here are some shifts that *might* show up as you move through the phases:

- **Cycle changes** (irregular, heavier, lighter, or completely erratic)
- **Sleep drama** (insomnia, night sweats, weird dreams)
- **Mood swings** that feel like puberty's angry older sister
- **Weight changes** that defy logic and your usual habits
- **Brain fog** that makes you forget what you walked into a room for
- **New food sensitivities**, bloating, or allergies that appear out of nowhere

Some symptoms will pass. Others may stick around. Either way, knowledge = power. You're not broken—you're evolving.

✧ **HOT TIP:** Start tracking your symptoms *now*, even if you're not sure what they mean yet. Use an app, a notebook, or a scrap of paper. Patterns will emerge. This is your data, and it can help you advocate for better care, better treatments, and a better quality of life.

1.3 HORMONAL HAVOC: UNDERSTANDING ESTROGEN, PROGESTERONE, AND MORE

If menopause had a villain origin story, it would start with your hormones pulling a vanishing act. But this isn't a Marvel movie—there's no single "bad guy." It's more like your body's internal orchestra suddenly loses its conductor and starts free-styling.

The primary divas in this hormonal drama? **Estrogen** and **progesterone**.

The Hormone Drop-Off

Before menopause, estrogen and progesterone are the backstage crew keeping things running: regulating your cycle, supporting mood, protecting your bones, helping you sleep, keeping your skin and vagina hydrated, and even helping your heart and brain work smoothly. You don't really notice them—until they start packing up and leaving the scene.

During perimenopause, these hormones don't just decline—they *fluctuate*, sometimes wildly. This rollercoaster is what causes many of the symptoms you may already be experiencing: hot flashes, anxiety, mood swings, and changes in sleep, libido, and cognition.

Estrogen drops = your internal thermostat goes haywire. Progesterone drops = your calming, stabilizing hormone exits stage left, and you're left with what feels like emotional whiplash.

The Other Hormones in the Mix

While estrogen and progesterone hog the spotlight, other hormones also affect how you feel:

- **Testosterone** (yes, women have it too) helps with energy, libido, and drive. It declines gradually and can leave you feeling flat or unmotivated.
- **Cortisol**, your stress hormone, can get louder during this time—especially if menopause is colliding with other life stressors (which, let's be honest, it usually is). High cortisol = more anxiety, more inflammation, less resilience.
- **Thyroid hormones** can also shift during this time. And when they're off, they can mimic or magnify menopausal symptoms.

This is why some people feel like their body is betraying them on multiple fronts. It's not in your head. It's in your *hormones*—and understanding them is the first step to working *with* your body, not against it.

So... Should You Get Your Hormones Tested?

Short answer: **maybe—but with the right expectations.**

A single hormone test isn't going to hand you a perfect diagnosis or a magic solution. Hormones fluctuate *daily*—especially during perimenopause—so one snapshot in time can be misleading.

That said, **tracking hormone levels over time**, alongside your symptoms, *can* provide valuable insights. It's especially helpful when you're working with a provider who understands perimenopause and can interpret the full picture.

Think of testing like using GPS during a road trip: one point on a map won't tell you much, but look at a bunch of points and that can help guide your next move.

My Experience with Testing

I was deep in the "WTF is happening to my body" phase when I decided to start tracking my hormones more intentionally. I asked my doctor for a full blood panel—yes, a fasting draw, super quick, usually covered by insurance. It didn't just include estrogen and progesterone—it gave me a bigger picture: thyroid function, inflammation markers, vitamin D (hello, bone health), blood sugar, and more.

At first, I tested every three months to see how things shifted. Now, I check in about twice a year. Reviewing those results alongside my symptoms has helped me connect the dots on this road trip that is menopause. It's not about perfection—it's about having a *conversation with your body* instead of being left in the dark.

✦ **HOT TIP:** Bring a copy of your symptom log or journal to your doctor's appointment. It gives your provider a richer picture than one blood test ever could.

1.4 THE EMOTIONAL LANDSCAPE: MOOD SWINGS AND MENTAL HEALTH

Let's talk about the part of menopause that doesn't get nearly enough airtime: the emotional whiplash.

One minute you're laughing at a meme. The next, you're crying in your car because you forgot your grocery list. Or you're in a full-blown rage spiral because someone loaded the dishwasher wrong. (Again.)

> "Mood regulation—irritability, weepiness, that short fuse—is one of the most common and most ignored early symptoms. It's easier to trigger those stronger emotions, and the lack of sleep just amplifies everything."
>
> — DR. BOURGEOIS, ND

These mood swings are not a personality flaw. They're not proof you're "losing it." They're a very real, very hormonal mindfuck brought to you by your good friend, **estrogen**.

What's Actually Happening

Estrogen plays a major role in regulating serotonin, one of the brain's mood-balancing chemicals. When estrogen levels start swinging, serotonin follows—and so do your emotions.

You might feel anxious for no reason.

Sad without warning.

Enraged over minor annoyances.

You may not even recognize yourself.

And that's terrifying.

But it's not just in your head.

It's chemical—and it's normal.

As Christina Cameli, CNM, points out:

> "We know that perimenopause increases the risk for depression, anxiety, and even eating disorders. It's not hypothetical—hormones and mental health are deeply connected."

How to Cope When the Ground Feels Shaky

There's no magic wand for emotional symptoms—but there *are* tools.

- **Mindfulness practices** like deep breathing, journaling, or even five quiet minutes in your car can offer real relief. It's not about achieving inner peace—it's about getting through the damn day with a little more ease.
- **Talk to someone.** A friend, a partner, a therapist. You're not alone, and you don't have to figure this out in isolation.
- **Check in with your provider.** Mental health deserves as much attention as physical health—especially now. If you're feeling constantly overwhelmed, flat, angry, or numb, speak up. There's no gold star for muscling through.

When Your Identity Feels Like It's Shifting Too

It's not just your emotions that are in flux—sometimes, it's your whole sense of self.

You might look in the mirror and feel disconnected from the face staring back. You might wonder what happened to the driven, vibrant, witty version of you. You might feel like everything familiar—your routines, your roles, even your confidence—is suddenly up for renegotiation.

You might even think, "How the hell did I get here?"

It's uncomfortable as hell. But it's also a chance.

This isn't a midlife crisis. It's a midlife *rewrite*. You get to reimagine how you spend your time, what lights you up, and which pieces of your identity you want to amplify—or let go of.

Now that is true power.

My Own Mental Reset

I've always told stories. I figured someday I'd write a book called *101 Stories of Ridiculous Risks, Dumb Decisions, and a Lot of Luck That My Mom Never Wanted to Hear About but is Now Because I Wrote a Book: The Illustrated Edition*.

Instead, I'm writing *this* book. Why? Because I finally reached the "fewer shits to give" phase of life. And let me tell you—it's glorious.

That mindset helped me stop worrying about whether I was doing menopause "right" and start doing what felt real.

One of the best moves I made early on? **Therapy.** Not because I was falling apart, but because I needed perspective. My therapist didn't give me a life overhaul—she suggested I add a few cozy pillows to my office couch.

I know. Pillows.

But those pillows turned my workspace into a little sanctuary. A place to pause, breathe, and remember that I get to *choose* how I show up—even on the messiest days.

Journaling Prompt:

What emotions have shown up most often for you lately? Are there moments when you've felt disconnected from yourself—or, on the flip side, surprisingly grounded? Jot down any emotional experiences from the past week, without judging or the urge to "fix" anything. Sometimes, naming what you're feeling is the first step to understanding and navigating it.

1.5 DEBUNKING MYTHS: SEPARATING FACT FROM FICTION

Menopause gets a bad rap—and not because of the symptoms, but because of the **bullsh*t narratives** we've absorbed about what it is and what it means.

Let's start here: **Menopause is not just about hot flashes and mood swings.** It's not the end of womanhood, relevance, or joy. You're adapting—beautifully, imperfectly, powerfully. And that's not scary—it's powerful.

Busting the Big Myths

Myth #1: Menopause = hot flashes and that's it.

Hot flashes might show up (and when they do, you'll know), but menopause affects way more than your thermostat. Sleep, focus, joints, libido, energy, confidence—it can touch every corner of your life. But it's different for everyone. Some folks feel off for a week. Others feel like their body has become a stranger. Both are real. Both are normal.

Myth #2: Menopause is the end of femininity.

Hard no. This is the beginning of something new—not the end of anything essential. Your femininity doesn't disappear. It deepens, strengthens, and becomes less about performance and more about truth. *Your* truth. You still get to be vibrant, sexy, opinionated, adventurous—whatever you decide that looks like.

Myth #3: Hormone Replacement Therapy (HRT) causes cancer.

This one is personal. When I first started navigating menopause, I *still* believed this. Like many people, I'd heard that HRT was dangerous—and never got the memo that those early 2000s headlines were based on misunderstood science.

Here's the truth: the **Women's Health Initiative (WHI)** study released in 2002 did suggest an increased risk of breast cancer with HRT, but that data was later reevaluated. The media panic didn't reflect the nuance: that the risk varies by age, health history, and type of HRT. For many women, especially those under 60 and within 10 years of menopause onset, **the benefits outweigh the risks**. That includes relief from hot flashes, bone protection, cardiovascular support, and more.

Bottom line: **HRT is not the villain.** It's a powerful option and deserves thoughtful, individualized discussion, not fear-based avoidance.

Why the Truth Matters

Misinformation makes people suffer. It keeps them in silence. It stops them from asking questions. When we shine light on the facts—on the *real* science—we make room for better decisions, improved care, and more connection.

You're not weak. You're not crazy. You're not alone. You're going through something deeply human. Let's stop whispering about it.

Trust Yourself—Especially in the Exam Room

You've heard me tell the story already—about the doctor who told me to try a box food diet and called it good. That moment lit a fire in me. Because here's the thing: **I deserve better. And you do too.**

If something doesn't feel right during a healthcare visit, listen to that inner voice. Ask more questions. Speak up. Push back. Or walk out. And if advocating for yourself feels hard? Bring someone who can be your voice, your support, or just your second set of ears.

✦ **HOT TIP: If a provider discourages you from bringing a support person, that's a red flag.** The right doctor wants you empowered, informed, and confident—not isolated.

Menopause Isn't Universal—But It Is Global

How menopause is experienced—and how it's framed—varies widely across cultures.

In some places, menopause is a rite of passage into wisdom and power. In others, it's seen as the beginning of decline. Those cultural lenses shape how we feel about ourselves. They shape what we expect—or fear. And they shape what kind of support we even think we deserve.

That's why it's so important to hear a range of stories, from a range of women. There's no one way to do menopause. There's only your way—and that should be enough.

Famous Faces, Real Talk

Some public figures are helping break the silence, too.

Naomi Watts experienced menopause at age 36 and spoke candidly about feeling isolated and unsupported. Now, she's using her platform to normalize the conversation and help other women feel less alone.

Michelle Obama shared her experience of hot flashes during a high-stakes political meeting and reminded millions of women that it's okay to talk about it out loud, without shame.

Want more truth? Start with these:

- *The Menopause Manifesto* by Dr. Jen Gunter
- *Menopausing* by Davina McCall & Dr. Naomi Potter
- *The Wisdom of Menopause* by Dr. Christiane Northrup

1.6 SOCIETAL STIGMAS AND BREAKING THE SILENCE

For too long, menopause has been kept in the shadows—treated like a taboo, a punchline, or something to endure quietly with a clenched jaw and a cardigan.

We've been taught to shrink as we age. To whisper instead of shout. To believe menopause is the end of our vitality, rather than the evolution of our power.

That silence? It's cost us. It has isolated us. And it's time to break it.

How We Got Here

Historically, menopausal women were often dismissed as unstable, hysterical, or unhinged. That stigma stuck—and media didn't help. Too often, we've been portrayed as irrational, overly emotional, or just plain irrelevant.

The result? A cultural script that says menopause = decline. That says we should disappear quietly. That says we should be ashamed of this transformation.

And most of us? We internalized it. We stopped talking. We powered through. We pretended we were fine.

The Power of Speaking Up

But here's the truth: every time one of us talks openly about menopause, we chip away at that silence. And we make it easier for someone else to speak, too.

I'll never forget standing center track at a roller derby bout, sweating my ass off, and telling a crowd of 500 people—and everyone watching on the live stream—that I was deep in menopause. Then I shouted out our sponsor, Menopause Northwest, and handed out co-branded fans to everyone dealing with hot flashes.

It was part PSA, part comedy set, and part community moment—and it worked. People *laughed, nodded,* and *raised their hands.* We created a connection. We helped women feel seen. In that sweaty room, surrounded by the energy of derby, we normalized menopause.

Modern Platforms, Real Connection

Thanks to social media, we now have megaphones in our pockets.

Whether you're posting TikToks, sharing Instagram stories, or quietly lurking in Facebook groups, *you're participating in the cultural shift.* Online communities and hashtags are helping women find each other, share symptoms, trade tips, and—maybe most importantly—realize they're not alone.

Not everyone needs to be loud. Some people just need to see someone else say, "Hey, I'm in it too." That's also activism.

Ways to engage:

- Post a comment or share a meme that hits home
- Follow creators who are keeping it real
- Join a group chat, a support circle, or a book club
- Just listen—and know you're part of something bigger

✦ **HOT TIP:** If talking publicly feels too vulnerable, start small. A heart emoji on someone else's menopause post is still part of the movement.

Leaders Who Are Loud and Proud

This movement isn't just grassroots—it's going global, thanks to some badass advocates with big platforms.

Dr. Jen Gunter is calling out junk science and misinformation with facts, feminism, and zero tolerance for BS.

Oprah Winfrey is talking openly about hormone therapy, brain fog, and the right to feel *good* in this chapter of life.

These women are helping shift the cultural narrative, reminding us that menopause is *not* a decline. It's a declaration.

1.7 THE POWER OF KNOWLEDGE: PREPARING FOR YOUR JOURNEY

Menopause can feel like a twisty, unfamiliar road, but having a map changes everything.

Knowledge is your GPS. It won't eliminate every pothole or detour, but it will keep you from feeling less alone, less overwhelmed, and a hell of a lot more confident. When you understand what's happening in your body, what's likely to come next, and what your options are, you stop reacting and start planning.

You're not walking blind—you're building your own damn toolkit.

Pack Your Tools (and Use Them Your Way)

This transition is about preparation, not perfection. When you approach it with curiosity and structure, you stop waiting for a breakdown and start building a strategy.

Here's what that looked like for me:

I started with the pain I couldn't ignore—**plantar fasciitis**—and the emotional weight I'd been carrying. So I found a therapist.

Then I started tackling the deeper shifts—**fluctuating hormones, food allergies, lack of motivation, and sleep disruption**. Once those were in motion, I began building strength. I upped my workouts, adjusted my supplements, dialed in my protein and fiber, and most recently added adaptogens.

It didn't happen all at once. It was layered and messy and deeply human. But the key? I kept moving forward. *Progress, not perfection.*

Speak Up, Build Your People

You're not meant to go through this alone.

Talking openly—with your doctor, your friends, your family, your coworkers—is one of the most powerful things you can do. It breaks shame, builds connection, and creates a ripple effect that helps *everyone*.

Start small. Tell one person what you're navigating. Ask for what you need. Keep inviting people in. You never know who's desperate for that same permission.

A New Chapter, Not the Last One

This moment in your life? It's not a conclusion—it's a shift. A chance to reset, reprioritize, and rethink what you want next.

We're just getting started. This chapter laid the groundwork. What's coming next will help you manage symptoms, explore treatments, and build a plan that actually fits your life.

So take a breath. You've already done the brave thing—you're showing up and learning. Now let's get into the good stuff.

Understanding the Menopausal Transition

KEY Takeaways

1. Perimenopause can start 5–10 years before your last period.
2. Hormone fluctuations and decline trigger early symptoms.
3. Tracking symptoms empowers smarter treatment and advocacy.

HOT TIPs

- 💎 Track 5 symptoms daily for 30 days to spot patterns.
- 💎 Use hormone testing as a tool, not a verdict.
- 💎 Mood swings = chemical shifts, not personality flaws.

ACTION ITEMS

- ☐ Download a symptom tracker app (Balance, MySysters) or use a notebook.
- ☐ Record 3 physical and 2 emotional symptoms daily for one month.
- ☐ List your top 3 weirdest symptoms to discuss at your next appointment.
- ☐ Share one symptom experience with a trusted friend or partner.

✦ Resources ✦

- Web: Menopause.org Symptoms
- Book: The Menopause Manifesto by Dr. Jen Gunter
- Instagram: @drmaryclaire
- Podcast: The Midlife Feast with Shirley Weir

NEXT UP — *Get ready to dive into symptom relief: cooling hot flashes, restoring sleep, lifting brain fog, and finding small daily hacks that change everything.*

2

MASTERING EVERYDAY SYMPTOM RELIEF

B*ecause You Shouldn't Have to Google "Why Do I Feel Like a Volcano With Rage Issues?"*

Welcome to the meat and potatoes (or tofu and quinoa, if that's your thing) of menopause: the symptoms. This is the part where things get real, fast. One day you're cruising along, and the next, you're crying in a Target parking lot because the air conditioning is broken, and they're out of your favorite sparkling water. Sound familiar? You're not alone.

Hot flashes, night sweats, mood swings, weight changes, insomnia, and the sudden, soul-sucking disappearance of your libido —these aren't signs you're losing your mind. They're signs your hormones are throwing a rave and didn't invite you to the DJ booth.

This chapter is your toolkit. Think of it like a fanny pack full of smart strategies, science-backed solutions, and a few spicy suggestions for riding out the menopause storm with style. You'll learn how to cool off (literally), sleep better, manage your moods like the emotionally intelligent goddess you are, and feel more connected to your body again—even the parts that feel like they've gone rogue.

You won't find shame here. Just support, laughter, and real-deal help. Menopause is a powerful transition, not a punishment. And while the symptoms may be loud and sometimes absurd (hello, ear ringing?!), they are manageable—with the right tools, mindset, and maybe a fan the size of a small jet engine.

Let's get into it. You've got this.

2.1 HOT FLASH HACKS: STAYING COOL UNDER PRESSURE

When your body decides to spontaneously combust—at the worst possible moment.

Picture this: You're mid-meeting, killing it, and suddenly a wave of heat crashes over you like a hormonal tsunami. Your face flushes, sweat trickles down your spine, and you're suddenly aware of every single layer of clothing you're wearing. Welcome to hot flashes—the menopause party crashers that always arrive uninvited and never bring snacks.

For many women, they're more than just uncomfortable. They're inconvenient, embarrassing, and make you wonder if your body is actively trying to sabotage you. But don't worry—you're not powerless. With a few clever tricks and small adjustments, you can cool things down and reclaim your calm.

Find Your Triggers (Even If You Love Them)

Identifying what sets off your hot flashes is key. But fair warning: some of them might sting. Spicy food? That was half your personality. Red wine? Your trusty dinner date. Stress? Well… good luck avoiding that.

I remember feeling personally attacked by my triggers. I'd always thrived under pressure, never met a jalapeño I didn't like, and proudly wore my life-of-the-party badge. So, when I realized these things were lighting the hormonal fire, I had a bit of an identity crisis. But acknowledging those triggers—and dialing some of them back—brought major relief.

Start keeping track of what you eat, drink, and do when a hot flash hits. A simple journal or even a few notes on your phone can help you connect the dots, or get the app Balance - Menopause & Hormones By Dr Louise Newson. Maybe it's your afternoon coffee. Or your late-night rewatch of *Yellowjackets*. Once you've got the pattern, you can decide what's worth minimizing (or at least timing better).

What to Do in the Moment

Sometimes the flash hits before you can say "deep breath." Here's how to ride it out with grace—or at least without panic:

- **Practice calming breathwork.** Inhale deeply through your nose, hold it, and exhale slowly through your mouth. I like to picture inhaling sparkly white mist and exhaling a cloud of black toxic energy. It weirdly helps.
- **Stash a fan or cooling mist in your bag.** Small, mighty, and a total lifesaver.
- **Stick a cold water bottle to your chest or neck.** Quick, direct relief. Bonus if it's straight from your freezer.

These aren't cure-alls, but they can turn a full-on meltdown into a manageable moment.

Dress Like the Goddess of Thermoregulation

Your wardrobe becomes part of your cooling toolkit. Breathable fabrics like cotton and linen are your best friends. And layers? Absolute game-changers. During my peak hot-flash era, I lived in cardigans—sweater on, sweater off, sweater back on—as if I were reenacting a fashion montage for one.

The drama even made its way to Zoom. One day, the flashes were so intense I ended up sitting in my bra mid-meeting. My Ops Manager, Nancy, texted, "Are you in your bra?" to which I replied, "Yep. Sometimes you've got to do what you've got to do." Menopause isn't always graceful, but it *is* real—and practicality wins. Don't worry my camera was pointed high enough up to not embarrass anyone.

Food That Cools You From the Inside

Some foods may help regulate your hormones naturally, especially those rich in phytoestrogens—plant compounds that gently mimic estrogen. You don't need to overhaul your whole diet, but sprinkling in these ingredients can help:

- Soy (tofu, edamame, soy milk)
- Flaxseeds and sesame seeds
- Chickpeas and lentils
- Apples, berries, pomegranates
- Broccoli, cauliflower, carrots
- Whole grains like oats, quinoa, and barley
- Healthy fats from nuts, avocados, and olive oil

If you're soy-sensitive, no problem. Flax, seeds, and legumes are still in your corner. And if you're not sure where to start, a nutritionist can help you tailor these swaps to your needs.

Cool Tech = Hot Flash Superpowers

Your environment matters, and so does your gear. Cooling pillows and mattress pads can make sleep more manageable. Wearable cooling tech—like neck fans or cooling jewelry—can bring real relief, even on the go. Plus, let's be honest: wearing a chic cooling necklace and having another woman say, "Wait, is that for *menopause?*" is its own kind of solidarity.

It's a sweaty sisterhood out here. And that moment of connection is sometimes the best thing to come from a hot flash.

You may not be able to avoid hot flashes entirely, but with a little sleuthing, a few tools, and the willingness to peel off your sweater (or shirt!) mid-Zoom, you can manage them like the cool, collected legend you are.

2.2 SLEEP SOLUTIONS: OVERCOMING INSOMNIA AND NIGHT SWEATS

Sleep, once a reliable and welcomed escape from the chaos of daily life, can suddenly become elusive during menopause. Insomnia and night sweats tag-team your nights, turning what used to be a peaceful recharge into a restless battle. Hormonal fluctuations are largely to blame—as estrogen and progesterone levels drop, they interfere with neurotransmitters that regulate your sleep cycle. The result? Your internal clock short-circuits. And just when you're finally drifting off, you're jolted awake by a flash of heat that leaves your sheets soaked and your mood wrecked.

To make matters worse, your brain—ever the overachiever—likes to join in the fun by spiraling into stress and anxiety mode just as your head hits the pillow. The daily pressures of life, now layered with the invisible load of changing hormones, amplify restlessness. Cue the 3 a.m. mental to-do list.

But the good news? There are practical ways to reclaim your rest. And none of them require you to become a zen monk or invest in blackout curtains made from unicorn hair.

Cool Down Your Sleep Space

A cooler environment can make a world of difference when you're battling night sweats. Whether it's turning down the thermostat, cracking a window, or investing in a personal fan, finding your ideal sleep temperature is a game-changer. I personally went through a whole fan journey—testing speeds, angles, and sound levels—until I hit my sweet spot (it's level two on my tower fan, oscillating 4 feet from me). I also started wearing my hair up to bed, which allowed the fan to actually reach my neck. Tiny shift, major impact.

If you share a bed, negotiating sleep temperature can be tricky (especially if your partner runs cold). I moved my bedtime an hour earlier so I could fall asleep without the heat battle, and honestly, it made everything better. My husband was happy to get on board once he noticed I wasn't waking up grumpy and sweating through the sheets. Everyone wins.

Build a Routine That Tells Your Brain, "It's Bedtime"

Creating a consistent wind-down ritual trains your brain to prepare for sleep. For me, that meant developing a nighttime self-care routine. It's nothing fancy—I brush and floss (OK, not nightly, let's be real), remove my makeup, wash my face, exfoliate or mask a couple times a week, then follow up with a serum and moisturizer. Am I finally using the expensive skincare products I hoarded for years? Yes. Do I feel smug about it? Also yes.

And if you're scrolling TikTok for skincare tips like I am, remember: don't trust the 22-year-olds. We all looked amazing at 22, even after three hours of sleep, too many vodka sodas, and last night's M.A.C. makeup. You're building a ritual for now —for your body, your skin, your peace.

Relax Your Mind, Not Just Your Muscles

Sometimes the physical environment is perfect, but your brain still refuses to shut up. That's where calming techniques can help flip the switch.

- **Deep breathing** can signal your nervous system that it's safe to rest. Inhale slowly through your nose, exhale through your mouth, and visualize stress leaving your body like a cloud of smoke.
- **Progressive muscle relaxation** involves tensing and releasing muscle groups one by one—feet to forehead—which helps your body power down.
- **Guided meditations** or sleep stories (via apps like Calm or Insight Timer) can gently distract your mind and lull you into rest.

One practice that's made a huge difference for me? Writing down the next day's top priorities before I get into bed. It tricks my brain into thinking everything is under control so it doesn't wake me up at 3 a.m. with an urgent reminder to buy toothpaste or finally reply to that email I've been avoiding for a week.

✥ **HOT TIP:** Can't sleep? Try a body scan meditation. It's a simple way to relax muscles and quiet racing thoughts—search YouTube or Calm for a free version.

And While We're at It...

This isn't a lifestyle lecture, but if you're regularly struggling with sleep, it's worth noticing a few things:

- Alcohol might *feel* like it helps you fall asleep, but it often wakes you up a few hours later.
- Caffeine lingers longer than we think, especially as our hormones shift. Cutting off coffee in the early afternoon can make a big difference.
- Screen time before bed—scrolling your phone, binging Netflix—can mess with melatonin production. Try switching to a book or podcast instead.

Again, you don't have to overhaul your life. But small changes add up.

When You've Tried It All and You're Still Exhausted

Sometimes, even when you're doing everything "right," sleep remains elusive. If that's your reality, it might be time to talk to a pro. We'll dig into medical and alternative options in later chapters, but a sleep study or consultation with specialists can uncover hidden issues and offer personalized support.

Your healthcare provider may suggest short-term medication, supplements, or other therapies. The key is to have an open, honest conversation and explore what aligns with your broader health goals. You are not alone, and you are not doing anything wrong—menopause sleep issues are *common*. Getting help isn't failure. It's strategy.

You deserve good sleep—not just to function, but to *feel* like yourself again. With a little curiosity, some environmental tweaks, and a willingness to experiment, you can reclaim your nights and start waking up feeling like you actually slept. Imagine that.

2.3 MOOD BALANCING ACT: EMOTIONAL WELL-BEING AND STABILITY

Menopause has a way of flipping your emotional switch without warning. One moment you're fine, the next you're crying because you dropped an egg (in this economy!). These shifts aren't just "in your head". They're wired into your hormones.

Estrogen helps regulate serotonin, the brain chemical responsible for mood and happiness. When estrogen dips, so can serotonin, leaving you more prone to mood swings, sadness, or irritability. Progesterone plays its part, too. When it's out of balance, anxiety can spike. Together, this hormonal cocktail can leave you feeling like a stranger in your own skin.

This chapter focuses on practical, non-medical strategies to help you ride those emotional waves. We'll get into medications, supplements, and alternative therapies in Chapter 4, and take a deeper dive into emotional and mental wellness—including therapy, identity shifts, and building long-term resilience—in Chapter 6. But here, we'll start with some everyday tools and mindset shifts you can use right now.

Mind Over Menopause: Cognitive and Reflective Tools

When your emotions feel like they're running the show, **Cognitive Behavioral Therapy with Mindfulness** (CBT-Ms) can help you take the wheel again. CBT-M strategies are all about identifying unhelpful thought patterns and gently rewiring them.

Let's say you catch yourself spiraling into worst-case thinking: "I'll never sleep again," "Everyone's mad at me," or "This meeting is going to ruin my career." CBT-M helps you pause, question the thought, and replace it with something more balanced—something rooted in reality instead of runaway hormones.

Journaling can also be powerful. Writing things down helps you track patterns, release built-up tension, and check whether your reaction actually matches the situation. These days, I've developed a little internal alarm that goes off when my emotions veer too far in one direction. If I feel overly anxious, weepy, or notice that the permanent grouch line on my forehead is extra deep, I pause and say out loud what's going on. It helps me name the feeling and figure out whether it's grounded in something real —or just hormones playing dress-up as a crisis.

Move Your Mood

Exercise is hands down one of the best mood stabilizers available—and no prescription is required. Physical movement releases endorphins, those glorious chemicals that can lift your spirits, calm anxiety, and make you feel more like yourself again.

Personally, if I skip more than a day, my mood starts to nosedive. A good sweaty session clears out the emotional "ick" and gets me back on track. My husband learned early on that suggesting I work out could either save his life or endanger it, depending on the tone. (Pro tip: "Wanna walk together?" goes over way better than "You should hit the gym.")

We'll get deeper into the benefits of exercise in Chapter 3, but if you're feeling emotionally off-kilter, movement can be your reset button.

Find Your Calm (Even If It Looks a Little Messy)

Mindfulness, breathing exercises, and gentle movement practices like yoga and tai chi can help soften the edges of emotional volatility. Mindfulness meditation encourages you to stay present, breathe deeply, and ride out the wave instead of letting it crash over you.

Now, full disclosure: the last time I tried yoga, I looked more like a disoriented baby giraffe than a peaceful goddess. So I started going to a functional stretch class instead. It's less intimidating, still centers my breath and body, and I don't feel like I'm about to topple into a potted plant.

The trick is finding something that works for *you*. It doesn't need to be elegant. It just needs to feel good and help you settle.

Create a Support Plan

Riding the mood rollercoaster is easier with a little backup. Let the people around you know how they can support you. That might mean space and a cup of tea, or a little loving nudge to go on a walk. The key is knowing what you need and communicating it—before the tears or the snapping or the spiral hit.

And don't underestimate the power of professional support. Seeing a therapist during this transition doesn't mean something's wrong—it means you're taking this seriously. I started therapy during menopause, and it felt like having a brilliant, calm co-pilot helping me steer through the fog. Whether it's traditional talk therapy, CBT-M, or a support group of women going through the same thing, external support can be a game-changer.

A Quick Reminder:

Here's what's normal (even if it doesn't *feel* normal):

- Mood swings that feel disproportionate
- Crying for no clear reason
- Unexpected anger or irritability
- Feeling anxious in situations that never used to faze you

You're not broken. You're adjusting in real time—and that's brave. You're navigating a major hormonal shift, and you deserve support, grace, and every tool available to help you feel more like yourself again.

2.4 WEIGHT WISDOM: TACKLING MENOPAUSAL WEIGHT GAIN

Menopausal weight gain has a sneaky way of showing up uninvited—like it's been waiting in the wings for this exact hormonal moment. But contrary to popular belief, it's not just about skipping a few workouts or indulging in dessert. The reasons run deeper, rooted in biology and the natural changes your body is navigating.

As estrogen declines, your metabolism slows, meaning you burn fewer calories at rest than you used to. Even if you're eating the same, your body might be storing more. Lower estrogen also changes how and where fat is stored, shifting it from your hips and thighs to your belly—an area associated with higher risks of heart disease and type 2 diabetes. And just to keep things interesting, insulin resistance often creeps in, making blood sugar harder to regulate and weight gain even more stubborn.

We'll dive more deeply into nourishing your changing body in the next chapter, but here's where we tackle weight head-on—

with practical tools, self-compassion, and no crash diets in sight.

Fuel First: Practical Dietary Shifts

One of the most effective strategies during menopause is surprisingly simple: focus on protein and fiber. These two powerhouses help keep you full, balance your blood sugar, and support your body's changing needs. For fiber, reach for beans, lentils, whole grains, and veggies. For protein, think chicken, fish, tofu, and eggs.

Cutting back on sugar and refined carbs is also key. These can spike insulin, encourage fat storage, and leave you feeling hungrier, faster. Instead, opt for complex carbs like sweet potatoes, oats, and quinoa—slow-burn energy that keeps you going without the crash.

And remember: this isn't about eliminating everything you love. It's about making *sustainable* changes that align with how you want to feel.

Your Relationship with Food Matters

This stage of your life is a perfect opportunity to get curious, not judgmental. Are you eating to nourish yourself? Or as a go-to response to stress, boredom, or burnout? No shame here—just awareness.

Menopause also comes with a powerful new filter: you stop giving as many fucks. That's a gift. It's not about restriction or punishment. It's about feeding your body in ways that support your energy, strength, and mood. Some days, that's a power bowl. Other days, it's a brownie. No guilt. No extremes. Just balance.

My Approach: Simpler, Smarter, Kinder

For me, ditching the all-or-nothing mindset changed everything. I aim for protein and fiber in every meal, and I give myself flexibility beyond that. I use social media for budget-friendly meal inspiration (because eating the same three things gets old fast) and focus on whole, minimally processed foods—no more obsessing over calorie caps or low-fat everything.

And yes, I still eat treats, but now I look for ones with some protein or fiber to keep me satisfied longer. That intentionality helps me enjoy food without spiraling into restriction or guilt.

Also: shoutout to an old friend—the *Lose It* app. Turns out, it has a setting perfect for menopause that highlights protein and fiber goals, which totally shifted how I track. It feels empowering, not punishing. And that makes all the difference.

Move Your Body, Build Your Strength

Exercise isn't just about burning calories. It's about *building capacity*—physically, mentally, and emotionally. Strength training is especially effective during menopause, helping preserve muscle mass, support metabolism, and protect bone density.

> "A lot of women think they're overweight when they're really just under-muscled. Strength training is essential because as estrogen declines, we naturally lose muscle and bone density. Lifting weights is the key to keeping your metabolism strong and preventing brittle bones."
>
> — EMILY HOWELL, WCS

Incorporating resistance workouts (squats, lunges, resistance bands) two to three times a week can have a huge impact. Cardiovascular movement—walking, biking, dancing, swimming—also supports heart health, mood, and energy levels. Aim for 150 minutes a week, but focus on what feels fun and sustainable. The best workout is the one you'll actually do.

Support Your Mindset Too

Weight gain during menopause is both physical and emotional. Set realistic goals that focus on *how* you feel, not just what you weigh. Celebrate progress in all forms: feeling stronger, sleeping better, having more energy, or simply being consistent.

Emotional eating can creep in during stressful moments, so try building alternative coping strategies.

- Go for a walk.
- Journal what you're feeling.
- Do a five-minute breathwork video.
- Call or text someone who gets it.
- Stretch or dance it out.
- Step outside and feel the air on your face.
- Anything that soothes you without triggering the shame spiral.

Let Go of the Scale as the Only Story

The number on the scale isn't the whole picture. It's one data point, not a reflection of your worth or effort. Menopause is an invitation to release old rules and redefine what health and confidence look like on *your* terms.

Perfection isn't the goal. You just need a plan that feels kind, doable, and aligned with where you are right now. When it comes to weight during menopause, the goal isn't shrinking. It's **strengthening**—your body, your habits, and your belief in yourself.

2.5 LIBIDO LIBERATION: REIGNITING INTIMACY AND CONNECTION

Menopause can change how your body responds to intimacy—but understanding those shifts gives you power, not limitation. This is not about giving up on pleasure; it's about reclaiming it in a new, informed, and empowered way.

As hormones shift, you may notice changes in your libido—and no, it's not just in your head. Estrogen plays a key role in vaginal health and sexual function, and as it declines, you might experience dryness, reduced sensitivity, or take longer to feel aroused. Testosterone levels, which support desire and sexual response, may also dip. Add in the usual suspects—fatigue, hot flashes, mood swings, disrupted sleep—and intimacy can start to feel less like fun and more like one more thing on your to-do list.

But you're not broken. You're evolving. And that means new tools, new communication, and yes, new opportunities for connection. We'll go deeper into relationships and emotional intimacy in Chapter 7, but for now, let's explore some practical ways to support your sexual health and satisfaction during menopause.

Start with Physical Comfort

One of the most common—and fixable—barriers is vaginal dryness. Over-the-counter lubricants and moisturizers can make a world of difference, turning painful encounters into comfortable, even enjoyable, ones. There are several types to explore:

- **Water-based lubricants**: Gentle, easy to clean, and great for most condoms and toys.
- **Silicone-based lubricants**: Long-lasting and ideal for reducing friction during sex.
- **Oil-based lubricants**: Good for external use, but not recommended with latex condoms.

If dryness persists or intensifies, low-dose vaginal estrogen (available as a cream, ring, or tablet) or DHEA (like Intrarosa) can restore moisture and elasticity. These localized treatments act directly on the tissues without affecting your whole hormonal system—and yes, they're safe and effective when used under medical guidance.

Increase Sensitivity and Pleasure

With decreased blood flow and thinner tissues, arousal might take more time—and more intention. Vibrators and clitoral stimulation can increase circulation and sensation. Arousal gels and warming lubricants may help as well, offering a boost in responsiveness that can rebuild confidence and connection.

Don't underestimate the power of pelvic floor exercises either. Strengthening those muscles improves sensation, boosts orgasmic response, and supports urinary health. If Kegels aren't cutting it (or you're not sure you're doing them right), consider using an app like Elvie Trainer or working with a pelvic floor physical therapist. This isn't just about sex—it's about reclaiming your comfort, confidence, and strength.

Create Space for Intimacy

Spontaneity might feel out of reach these days, but intention is just as sexy. Scheduling intimate time doesn't have to feel clinical; it can be a shared ritual. Think warm baths, sensual massage, music, low lighting, laughter. These cues help your body shift from "task mode" to "connection mode."

Treat this time as something sacred—a pause from daily chaos and a chance to reconnect. When you create space for intimacy, your body learns to follow your lead.

When You Need More Support

If you're still feeling stuck, it's time to talk. A sexual health specialist can help you find solutions tailored to your needs— whether that's hormonal, emotional, or relational. Therapy, workshops, books, and online courses can all offer new tools for navigating this next phase of sexual health.

The bottom line? Talk about it. Talk until it gets less awkward. Talk until you find solutions. The more we normalize these conversations, the more we reclaim agency and joy in our bodies.

✦ **HOT TIPs:**

- **Lubricant layering**: Combine silicone for lasting glide and water-based for gentle comfort—it's like the conditioner and leave-in of lube.
- **Painful sex is treatable**: Don't tough it out. If something hurts, stop. Talk to a menopause specialist. There are real solutions.
- **Explore pelvic floor therapy**: It's not just for post-birth recovery. These specialists can help with sensation, confidence, and function at every age.

Embrace the Shift

Reigniting intimacy during menopause isn't about going back to how things were—it's about moving forward into what's possible. By addressing physical discomfort, exploring new ways to experience pleasure, and working with your body instead of against it, you can rediscover a version of intimacy that feels grounded, authentic, and deeply satisfying.

This is your permission slip to prioritize pleasure, connection, and confidence—on your own terms.

2.6 LESSER-KNOWN SYMPTOMS: IDENTIFYING AND MANAGING SURPRISES

Hot flashes and night sweats get all the airtime, but let's be real—menopause is sneakier than that. It's not just a handful of well-known symptoms; it's a full-body experience filled with twists, turns, and side effects no one warned you about. That's partly because we simply haven't studied menopause enough. Some symptoms haven't even made it into the textbooks yet. But that doesn't mean they aren't real—or that you're not experiencing them.

Talking about the weird stuff matters. It helps break the stigma, get people into menopause care sooner, and most importantly, makes you feel a little less alone when your knees ache, your favorite meal betrays you, and you cry in the cereal aisle for no clear reason.

So let's shine a light on the strange and unexpected. Here's a rundown of the lesser-known (but totally normal) symptoms that can show up during menopause—and what you can do about them.

Achy Joints: The Snap, Crackle, Pop of It All

One day you're walking down the stairs and realize your body sounds like a percussion section. Joints that once worked like a dream now creak and complain, even if you're still in your 40s. What gives?

Estrogen plays a role in keeping inflammation at bay. As it drops, joint pain can sneak in—especially in your knees, hips, hands, and back. Omega-3 supplements helped me a lot, and so did daily movement, even if it was just a stretch or a walk. Think of it like WD-40 for your body: motion keeps things running smoother.

Hair Thinning and Skin Changes: The Great Moisture Heist

You may wake up one day wondering, "Was my hair always this... sparse?" Or feel like your skin has suddenly gone from plump and radiant to dry and dull. Yep, that's menopause messing with collagen, hydration, and circulation.

This is your cue to invest in skin and hair care that actually *feels* good. Slather on the serums, get that scalp massager, and embrace whatever helps you look in the mirror and say, "Okay, still got it."

Food Sensitivities: When Your Favorite Meals Betray You

Here's a curveball I did *not* see coming—developing new food sensitivities in my 40s. I started noticing that I just didn't feel good after eating. Nothing major at first—just bloated, sluggish, uncomfortable. But it kept happening, and I couldn't pinpoint why.

The very first time I met with Dr. Bourgeois, my naturopath, I brought it up. I told her I didn't feel good more often than I *did*, especially after meals, and that something felt off. She didn't brush it aside or chalk it up to aging. Instead, she ordered a full food sensitivity blood panel. That test revealed a cascade of heightened sensitivities: peanuts (which I already suspected), but also wheat, soy, and corn. All the things I was eating regularly.

It's a testament to this truth: **write it down and share it all with your doctor—even the stuff that seems minor or unrelated.** If I hadn't mentioned how I felt after eating, I might still be muddling through, thinking that constant discomfort was "just life now."

Once I had my results, I went cold turkey. My doctor was surprised (and thrilled) that I made the shift so quickly—but honestly, the results were immediate. I thought it would mostly help my stomach, but the real magic? My joint pain decreased dramatically. I felt lighter, clearer, more like myself. Within a week, I was sleeping better, moving easier, and waking up without that "everything hurts" fog.

The hardest part? Giving up tacos and beer. (I still remember the last time I had them—March 2023. We had a good run.) And eating out can feel like navigating a glutenous, soy-laced minefield. But the trade-off? Absolutely worth it. I feel more in control of my health, deeply in tune with what my body is asking for, and *sixty pounds lighter*!

Changes in Body Odor: Sniff Happens

Here's one they don't put in the pamphlet: menopause can mess with how you smell. Your natural scent might change thanks to shifting hormones, and suddenly, your go-to deodorant isn't cutting it. You're not imagining it—and you're definitely not alone.

Natural deodorants, breathable fabrics, and antibacterial soap can help. So can a sense of humor. Because if you're going to break a sweat just trying to park your car, you might as well laugh about it.

Alcohol Intolerance: The Betrayal Is Real

I used to handle four drinks like a champ. These days? Menopause has changed the game. Some nights I can still rally and have a blast. Other times, just a couple drinks hit *way* harder than expected—and suddenly I'm the one Irish-exiting before the DJ even gets going. It's not about drinking less out of guilt or pressure. It's just that alcohol hits differently now, thanks to hormone fluctuations and shifts in liver metabolism.

I've started making mocktails while I cook, and on nights I skip alcohol completely, I *definitely* sleep better. I still go out, I still love a wild night, and I still drink—but I pay closer attention to how I feel. I also make a deal with myself: if I'm drinking, I've already committed to making it to the gym the next morning. That little promise helps me keep things in check... most of the time.

Brain Fog: Wait, What Were We Talking About?

You walk into a room and forget why. You trail off mid-sentence like your brain just hit pause. It's not early dementia—it's hormones. That foggy feeling is incredibly common.

What helps: omega-3s, sleep, movement, reducing stress, and laughing about it instead of panicking. Also: post-it notes, alarms, and phone reminders. So many reminders.

Tingling Extremities: Not Just a "Slept Weird" Thing

Pins and needles in your hands and feet? Sometimes it's a nerve thing, sometimes circulation, but in menopause, it can be hormonal too. If it's new, persistent, or worrying, definitely check with your doc. But if it comes and goes, just know: you're not alone in feeling like your limbs are trying to send you secret Morse code.

Digestive Drama: Your Gut's New Mood

One day you can eat anything. The next? Bloating, gas, constipation—or all three at once. *Hooray!* Hormonal changes affect gut motility, and suddenly your digestion is like, "Yeah, we're doing things differently now."

Drink water, eat fiber, take your probiotics, and maybe slow down at meals. Menopause is the perfect time to learn how to chew slowly (finally).

Listen, Adapt, and Talk About It

These symptoms may not all show up for you—but some might. And if they do, you're not crazy. You're not "just getting older." You're going through a massive physiological shift. And the more we talk about it, the easier it gets.

Regular checkups help, but so does texting a friend and saying, "Is your left elbow buzzing for no reason too?" That connection is powerful—and it could help someone else recognize they've entered perimenopause, too.

Mastering the Mystery

Menopause isn't just a list of symptoms to "deal with." It's an opportunity to get to know your body in a new way, build resilience, and rewrite the rules for how you want to feel.

So here's your reminder: You're not falling apart. You're adjusting, evolving, and figuring things out in real-time. And that's strength, not weakness.

You've got this. Weird symptoms and all.

Wrapping Up Chapter 2

Menopause is a full-body, full-life transformation. From joint pain to brain fog, disrupted sleep to shifting libido, every surprise your body throws at you is a chance to get curious, get proactive, and get back in the driver's seat. And now? You've got tools.

This chapter was all about tackling symptoms with practical, everyday strategies—adjusting your environment, your routines, and your mindset. You've started building a foundation, and this is just the beginning.

In the chapters ahead, we'll go deeper into **how to support your body and mind through this transition and beyond**. We'll explore **nutrition and lifestyle**, dig into **medical and alternative therapies**, unpack **emotional and mental wellness**, and dive into **relationships, identity, and personal transformation**.

Because mastering your symptoms is important—but so is feeling strong, supported, and fully yourself in this new chapter of life.

Let's keep going. It only gets better from here.

Mastering Everyday Symptom Relief

KEY Takeaways

1. Hot flashes, night sweats, and mood shifts are hormone-driven.
2. Hydration, sleep, and movement help manage symptom intensity.
3. Symptoms vary wildly—your experience is valid and adaptable.

HOT TIPs

- 💎 Booze, spicy food, and stress can cause hot flashes.
- 💎 Cool your sleep space to 68°F for night sweat relief.
- 💎 Practice 4-7-8 breathing to calm anxiety and hot flashes.

ACTION ITEMS

- ☐ Track what triggers hot flashes for one week.
- ☐ Set a nightly 'tech-off' alarm 1 hour before bed.
- ☐ Journal the top 3 symptoms disrupting your daily life.
- ☐ Practice deep breathing, stretching, or meditation before sleep.

✦ Resources ✦

- App: Balance Menopause by Dr. Louise Newson
- Book: Next Level by Stacy Sims
- Instagram: @drjengunter
- Podcast: Hit Play Not Pause with Selene Yeager

NEXT UP — *Chapter 3 tackles nutrition, exercise, hydration, and fueling your midlife powerhouse body—no crash diets, just strength.*

3

NOURISHING YOUR BODY: NUTRITION AND LIFESTYLE

Imagine standing in your kitchen—a place where so many moments of your life have unfolded. From family dinners to late-night snacks, it's been the backdrop to countless memories. Now, it's where you begin a new chapter: menopause. This stage is about fueling your body for **strength, balance, and long-term health.**

3.1 NUTRITIONAL NEEDS: FEEDING YOUR CHANGING BODY

If there's one dietary shift every woman in perimenopause and menopause should prioritize, it's this: **Increase protein and fiber in every single meal.** These two nutrients are absolute game-changers for stabilizing blood sugar, preserving muscle mass, improving digestion, and keeping your metabolism steady.

While many general health experts recommend getting 0.45 to 0.68 grams of protein per pound of body weight per day, menopause coaches like Emily Howell suggest pushing those levels higher for optimum health during menopause especially when focusing on building muscle to protect our bones and boost our metabolism!

"Most women are severely under-eating protein. We need 0.8 to 1 gram per pound of body weight to build muscle and keep metabolism strong. Nutrition should fuel your body, not punish it." — Emily Howell, *WCS*

The Non-Negotiables: Protein and Fiber

✓ **Protein** is essential for retaining lean muscle, supporting metabolism, and keeping you full longer—especially as hormonal changes make it easier to gain fat and harder to maintain muscle. Without enough protein, your body loses muscle more quickly, which can lead to a slower metabolism, decreased strength, and a higher risk of injury.

- **Protein-Rich Foods:** Chicken, fish, eggs, Greek yogurt, tofu, tempeh, lentils, and lean beef.

✓ **Fiber** helps regulate blood sugar, supports gut health, reduces bloating, and keeps cholesterol in check—key factors as your metabolism shifts. It also feeds the good bacteria in your gut, which plays a role in hormone regulation and mood stabilization.

- **Fiber Powerhouses:** Vegetables, beans, berries, whole grains, flaxseeds, and chia seeds.

Every time you eat, ask yourself: Where's my protein? Where's my fiber? This simple habit ensures you're nourishing your body properly, without drastic restrictions.

✧ **HOT TIP:** Your body can't store protein for later use. That means if you're skipping it at breakfast or lunch, your muscles go hours without the nutrients they need to stay strong. **Aim for 20-30g of protein per meal** to keep your body fueled and actively preserving muscle.

Fiber needs water to do its job! If you start increasing fiber but don't drink enough water, you might end up feeling bloated or sluggish instead of energized. **Aim for at least half your body weight in ounces of water per day** to keep digestion running smoothly.

By making protein and fiber the foundation of your diet, you set yourself up for steady energy, balanced hormones, and long-term health. Now, let's break down the other key nutrients your body needs to thrive during menopause.

The Big Three: Calcium, Vitamin D, and Omega-3s

When I first learned that menopause increases the risk of osteoporosis and heart disease, it hit me hard. It wasn't just a theory; it was personal. A family friend broke her hip in her late 60s, and while she eventually recovered, it was a long and painful process. I remember thinking, *I don't want that to be me.* That's when I started taking calcium and vitamin D seriously—not just as buzzwords in a health ad, but as critical players in my long-term health.

Incorporating these nutrients into your diet is vital. As estrogen levels decline, they take some of their protective benefits with them, particularly for your bones and heart. Without enough calcium, bones weaken over time, increasing the risk of fractures. Without sufficient vitamin D, your body can't absorb calcium properly,making supplementation or fortified foods even more important—especially if you live in a place with limited sunlight.

And then there's omega-3 fatty acids, which reduce inflammation, protect heart health, and may even support brain function and mood stabilization. Since menopause brings a higher risk of cardiovascular disease, incorporating omega-3-rich foods is one of the smartest long-term strategies for keeping your heart healthy.

Where to Get These Nutrients

Calcium – Supports strong bones and prevents fractures.

- Dairy products: Milk, cheese, yogurt
- Fortified plant milks: Almond, soy, oat
- Leafy greens: Kale, collard greens, broccoli

Vitamin D – Enhances calcium absorption and supports bone health.

- Fortified foods: Orange juice, cereals
- Fatty fish: Salmon, sardines
- Supplements (especially in winter or for those with low sun exposure)

Omega-3 Fatty Acids – Support heart health, brain function, and may help stabilize mood.

- Fatty fish: Salmon, mackerel
- Plant-based sources: Flaxseeds, walnuts, chia seeds

✦ **HOT TIP:** Calcium and vitamin D work as a team. Without enough vitamin D, your body absorbs only a fraction of the calcium you consume. If you're not getting **at least 15 minutes of direct sunlight daily,** consider adding a vitamin D3 supplement.

Not all calcium supplements are created equal. Some forms, like calcium carbonate, need to be taken with food for optimal absorption, while calcium citrate can be taken anytime. If you experience bloating or digestive discomfort with calcium, switching to a different type can make a big difference.

By prioritizing these three powerhouse nutrients, you're protecting your bones, heart, and brain for the long haul—so you can keep moving, thinking, and thriving through menopause and beyond.

Whole Grains: Fiber, Energy, and Metabolic Stability

If you've ever felt like your metabolism has betrayed you during menopause, you're not alone. The afternoon slump is real. I used to reach for coffee and a sugary snack, only to crash hard an hour later. The fix? Prioritizing whole grains and fiber.

Whole grains are fiber powerhouses that stabilize blood sugar, improve digestion, and keep you feeling full longer. During menopause, when hormonal changes can spike cravings and slow metabolism, fiber becomes essential for keeping energy levels steady, preventing weight gain, and supporting gut health.

Fiber-Rich Whole Grains to Focus On

- **Quinoa** – A complete protein and fiber combo, perfect as a base for stir-fries, salads, or power bowls.
- **Oats** – Loaded with soluble fiber to support gut health and digestion; top with berries and Greek yogurt for the ultimate balanced breakfast.
- **Brown Rice** – A hearty, fiber-rich grain that pairs perfectly with lean proteins and roasted veggies.
- **Farro & Barley** – Great for soups and salads, offering

chewy texture and slow-digesting fiber to keep you satisfied longer.

If you're not used to eating much fiber, increase it slowly. Adding too much too fast can lead to bloating and discomfort. Start with one fiber-rich swap per day and build from there.

Making whole grains a daily habit keeps your metabolism stable and your energy strong, so you feel fueled rather than fatigued.

Leafy Greens: More Than Just a Side Dish

Leafy greens are loaded with magnesium and iron to support muscle function, red blood cell production, and energy levels. They also help combat fatigue, a common companion during menopause.

Many women in menopause experience low energy due to iron deficiency or magnesium depletion, both of which are found in abundance in leafy greens. Magnesium also plays a key role in stress reduction, muscle relaxation, and sleep quality—all areas that can take a hit during menopause.

How to Get More Greens in Your Day:

- **Kale Caesar salad** with a squeeze of lemon for extra vitamin C (which helps with iron absorption).
- **Spinach blended into your morning smoothie** for a hidden health boost.
- **Swiss chard sautéed with garlic** as a simple yet satisfying side dish.
- **Collard greens used as wraps** instead of tortillas for a fiber-packed alternative.
- **Arugula tossed into grain bowls** or omelets for a peppery kick and extra nutrients.

Don't love raw greens? No problem. Lightly sautéing or blending them into sauces and soups still retains most of the nutrients while making them easier to digest.

Choosing nutrient-rich foods is about more than just filling your plate—it's about creating a diet that supports your overall health and well-being. A daily dose of leafy greens can boost energy, improve digestion, and support long-term vitality.

Common Deficiencies to Watch For

Menopause can disrupt your body's nutritional balance, leading to deficiencies that leave you feeling sluggish, foggy, and off-kilter. Recognizing and addressing these gaps can be life-changing— often, small dietary changes or supplements make a huge difference in energy, mood, and overall well-being.

Iron Deficiency Anemia

I'll never forget the winter when I couldn't seem to get warm, no matter how many layers I wore. I felt drained, dizzy, and perpetually cold. It turned out I was iron-deficient—a common issue for women in menopause.

Since iron is critical for oxygen transport in the blood, low levels can cause fatigue, dizziness, cold extremities, and brain fog. This often results from heavy periods leading up to menopause or a reduced intake of iron-rich foods post-menopause.

I quickly learned that adding iron-rich foods to my diet made a noticeable difference in my energy and focus. I started incorporating lentils and chickpeas into hearty stews, sautéing spinach with olive oil and sea salt, and choosing fortified cereals topped with fresh fruit. Within weeks, I felt more alert and less drained, especially in the afternoons when I used to hit a wall of exhaustion.

✦ **HOT TIP:** Pair **iron-rich foods** (like **greens**) **with vitamin C sources** (like **oranges, bell peppers, or tomatoes**) to **enhance absorption** and maximize benefits.

Vitamin B12 Deficiency

B12 is another nutrient that caught me off guard. I started forgetting things—appointments, groceries, even my neighbor's name. It wasn't until my doctor ran blood work that I realized my B12 levels were low.

Vitamin B12 is essential for:

- **Energy production**
- **Brain function and memory**
- **Balance and nervous system health**

Since B12 is primarily found in animal-based foods, deficiencies are more common in vegetarians and vegans and in people with poor absorption issues, which can occur naturally with age.

Once I knew I needed more B12, I started small: grilled salmon or scrambled eggs for breakfast, fortified plant-based milks for dairy-free options, and nutritional yeast sprinkled on popcorn for a cheesy, B12-packed boost. I also began taking a B12 lozenge as part of my morning routine, and the improvement was almost immediate—clearer thinking, better memory, and a noticeable boost in energy.

✦ **HOT TIP:** If you're feeling off and can't quite pinpoint why, ask your doctor to run a full nutrient panel, including iron and B12. Deficiencies are often easy to correct with small dietary changes or targeted supplements, and the improvement in energy and mental clarity can be dramatic.

Meal planning isn't just about saving time and money—it's about setting yourself up for success, energy, and balance every single day. With the right prep and smart choices, you can eliminate the stress of last-minute meals, stay on track with protein- and fiber-rich options, and make eating healthy feel effortless.

I used to think meal planning was just for hyper-organized people with color-coded spreadsheets. But once I started doing it—even in the simplest way—my energy levels, digestion, and food choices improved dramatically. Taking just a few minutes to plan meals for the week meant fewer impulse decisions, less takeout, and way more meals that actually left me feeling good.

Plan Like a Pro

The best meal planning method is the one that works for you. For me, **Sundays are meal-planning day.** I take stock of what's in my fridge, jot down meals for the week, and make a precise grocery list so I don't end up buying random items I don't need. This helps me:

- **Use what I already have** (less waste, more savings).
- **Avoid last-minute takeout** when I'm too tired to cook.
- **Make sure every meal includes protein and fiber** to keep my energy steady.

✦ **HOT TIP:** In The One Life Planner, I map out my weekly meals, workouts, and goals, helping me stay focused on intentional eating and movement. Having a dedicated space for planning makes all the difference.

Batch Cooking for Effortless Meals

If you have nutrient-dense, protein- and fiber-packed meals ready to go, you'll always have a nourishing option no matter how hectic your day gets. This doesn't mean spending an entire Sunday cooking—just making a few things ahead can be a total game-changer.

One of my go-to strategies? Making a big pot of soup filled with veggies, lean protein, and fiber-rich beans or grains. It reheats beautifully and saves me from scrambling for a meal when I'm hungry. I also love roasting a tray of vegetables—sweet potatoes, Brussels sprouts, and peppers—so I can toss them into bowls, wraps, or salads throughout the week. And having pre-cooked proteins like grilled chicken, baked tofu, or hard-boiled eggs on hand ensures I never miss my protein goals.

Smart Snacking = No More Energy Crashes

Snacks should work **for** you, not against you. Keeping nutritious, grab-and-go options on hand helps prevent sugar crashes and mindless snacking. I always make sure my snacks pair protein with fiber for steady energy and satiety. Some of my go-tos:

- Almonds + apple
- Hummus + raw veggies
- Greek yogurt + chia seeds
- Hard-boiled eggs + a handful of berries

The Power of Proactive Planning

Meal planning is about freedom, not restriction. By taking a little time to plan, you ensure:

- **Balanced, nutrient-dense meals** that fuel your body.
- **Less decision fatigue**—you know what's for dinner before you're starving.
- **More consistency,** leading to **better energy, digestion, and hormone balance.**

Your Menopause Nutrition Mindset Shift

Menopause is a season of transformation, and the way you nourish your body can make all the difference. Think of your plate as your toolkit, filled with ingredients that empower you to feel strong, vibrant, and in control.

Small, intentional changes add up fast, so why not start today? Plan one protein- and fiber-packed meal for tomorrow and set yourself up for success!

"Eat Me": A cheeky cheat sheet to keep your meals protein- and fiber-forward.

Want a quick reminder to stick to protein and fiber? I created this downloadable "Eat Me" cheat sheet to make it easier. You can find it—along with all the other free resources mentioned in this book— www.menopauseunicorn.com

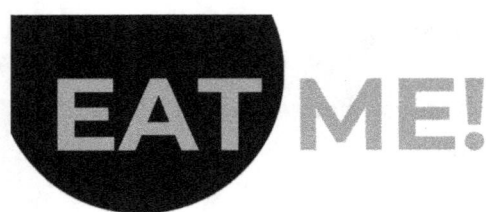

Protein

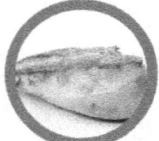
Chicken

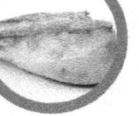
Greek Yogurt

Fiber

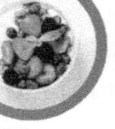
Greens

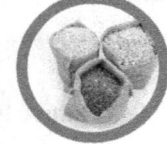
Whole Grains

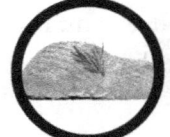
Fish

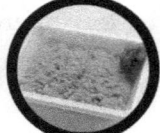
Turkey

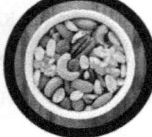
Nuts

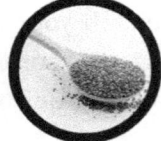
Chia Seeds

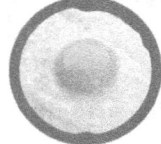
Eggs

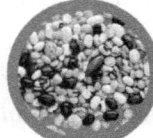
Beans & Lentils

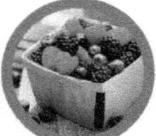
Berries

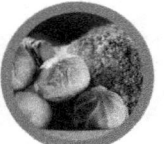
Brussels & Broc

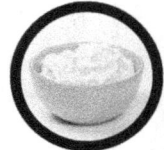
Cottage Cheese

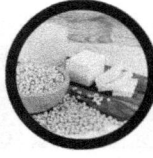
Soy

Don't forget The Big 3:
Calcium, Vitamin D, and Omega-3s

Download this at menopauseunicorn.com

3.2 EXERCISE ESSENTIALS: STAYING ACTIVE AND STRONG

Picture starting your day with an invigorating walk around the block, the crisp morning air filling your lungs and your thoughts untangling with each step. Exercise during menopause isn't just about movement—it's a lifeline. It's a natural mood booster, a stress reliever, and a powerful tool for regaining strength and control when your body is going through profound changes.

When you move your body, endorphins—the brain's **feel-good chemicals**—flood your system, lifting your mood and easing anxiety. But the benefits go far beyond mental well-being. Regular exercise is essential for:

- **Protecting your bones** – Strength training and weight-bearing exercises help prevent osteoporosis and maintain bone density.
- **Preserving muscle mass** – Muscle loss accelerates during menopause, so resistance training is non-negotiable for maintaining strength and metabolism.
- **Supporting heart health** – Cardiovascular exercise keeps your heart strong and resilient, reducing the risk of heart disease.
- **Improving balance & coordination** – Functional exercises help prevent falls and keep you steady on your feet.
- **Boosting metabolism & preventing weight gain** – Regular movement helps combat the hormonal shifts that make fat storage easier and muscle retention harder.

Most fitness professionals will tell you strength training is vital during menopause, including Emily Howell, who emphasizes the importance of working out smarter: more intensity, less volume, and more recovery. I live by this!

But I also believe in the golden rule: **The best workout is the one you'll actually do.** Let's build your personal menopause movement plan, one step at a time.

Step 1: Find Your Movement Mojo

Exercise is about feeling **alive, energized, and strong.** The key to consistency is choosing activities that you actually enjoy—because if you don't love it (or at least like it), you won't stick with it.

Here's how to build a menopause-friendly movement plan that works for YOU:

- **Strength Training** – Retains and builds muscle mass, supports bone density, and improves metabolism. Try bodyweight exercises, resistance bands, dumbbells, or weight machines.
- **Low-Impact Cardio** – Great for heart health and easy on the joints. Try swimming, cycling, rowing, or brisk walking.
- **High-Intensity Interval Training (HIIT)** – Quick, efficient, and boosts endurance. Try short bursts of squats, lunges, or jump rope with rest intervals.
- **Mobility & Stretching** – Keeps joints limber and reduces stiffness. Try yoga, Pilates, or dynamic stretching routines.
- **Social Sweat Sessions** – Exercising with friends makes it fun and keeps you accountable. Try a weekend hike, a dance class, or a walking catch-up with a friend.

For me, I mix strength training, HIIT, and functional stretching every week—it's what makes me hum. The variety keeps me energized, and I love incorporating movement into social time. A two-to-three-mile hike with a friend beats sitting in a coffee shop any day.

Step 2: Start Small—But Start Now

You don't need to overhaul your life overnight. Small, consistent changes build powerful habits.

- **Begin with 10 minutes a day.** A quick stretch, a brisk walk, or a few bodyweight exercises can jumpstart your routine.
- **Sneak movement into your day.** Take the stairs, park farther away, do 10 jumping jacks per hour, or do squats while brushing your teeth.
- **Commit to 3x per week.** Pick three workouts that feel doable and schedule them like non-negotiable appointments.
- **Track your wins.** Use a simple journal or app to stay motivated and watch your progress add up.

✦ **HOT TIP:** Sometimes you don't feel like working out and you can' tell if you're just not in the mood or if your body actually needs rest. Throw your workout gear on and commit to 5 minutes. 95% of the time, you keep going.

Step 3: Make Tech Work for You

Why not let AI and digital tools be your personal trainer, accountability partner, and motivation booster? Whether you need customized workouts, tracking tools, or a way to stay inspired, tech makes it easier than ever to stay on track.

AI-Generated Workouts: Your Personal Trainer on Demand

Recently, I used AI to build a **50-minute, full-body, low-impact strength workout** tailored to accommodate my recovering Achilles. The result? My workout crew and I sweated, smiled, and stayed pain-free, burning over **450 calories** with heart rates between **125–155 bpm**. AI coaching is real—and effective.

✔ **Try It:** Apps like Future, Fitbod, and Kemtai use AI to create personalized workouts that adapt to your fitness level and goals.

Social Media Fitness Trainers: Find Your People

Instagram and TikTok are goldmines for free, high-quality workouts—from strength training to yoga and dance cardio. Finding a trainer whose energy and approach resonate with you is a game-changer.

✔ **Try It:** Follow trainers who inspire you, save their workouts, and create a dedicated playlist of go-to routines.

✦ **HOT TIP:** Engage with your favorite trainers—comment on their videos, join their challenges, and use their content for motivation. **Feeling part of a community makes consistency so much easier.**

All-in-One Life & Fitness Planning: The One Life Planner

This is where the magic happens. I use The One Life Planner to organize everything:

- **Weekly meal planning** (so I actually eat nourishing food).
- **Mapping out workouts** (because consistency wins).
- **Setting goals** (big and small, on my vision board).
- **Tracking intentional conversations & gratitude** (because mindset matters).

Whether you prefer pen-and-paper or digital, having one central place to plan your workouts, meals, and goals keeps you focused, inspired, and on track for long-term success.

✓ **Try It:** Writing down workouts before the week starts makes it far more likely you'll follow through.

Track Your Progress Digitally

Traditional fitness tracking apps are great, but there are also modern tools that sync effortlessly with your lifestyle:

- **Habit-Tracking Apps:** Streaks, Habitica, or Notion to build momentum.
- **Wearables & Smartwatches:** Oura Ring, WHOOP, or Apple Watch to track workouts, recovery, and sleep.
- **Goal-Tracking Dashboards:** Notion, Evernote, or Trello to visualize progress and stay motivated.
- **Music & Motivation Playlists:** Spotify & Apple Music workout playlists for an energy boost.

Technology has made it easier than ever to stay active, track your progress, and stay accountable. Experiment with different tools, find what fits your lifestyle, and turn fitness into a natural, seamless part of your life.

Step 4: Build Exercise Into Your Life

Exercise isn't just a task—it can be woven into your daily routine in ways that feel effortless and enjoyable. The more movement becomes a natural part of your day, the less it feels like an obligation—and the more it becomes a built-in energy boost.

Think about movement as something you *get* to do, not something you *have* to do. It doesn't always have to be a structured workout. Everyday activities can add up to meaningful movement that keeps your body strong and your mind clear.

- **Quick Home Workouts** – Short, effective routines at home can be just as impactful as hour-long gym sessions. A 10-minute strength session or a few mobility exercises before bed still count!
- **Active Commuting** – If your destination is within walking or biking distance, take the opportunity to move instead of drive. Even small choices—like parking farther away or taking the stairs—add up over time.
- **Walking Meetings** – Whether on a work call or catching up with a friend, walk while you talk. You'll move more without even thinking about it.
- **Workout Rewards** – Treat yourself to new gear, a fun class, or a self-care moment when you hit your movement goals. A little incentive can go a long way.

By integrating movement into your daily life, exercise stops feeling like a chore and becomes second nature. The goal is to stay active in a way that feels good for you, every day.

Step 5: Safety First—Protect Your Body

Your body is changing, and safety matters more than ever. Mobility is a life-long goal. Before jumping into a new routine, make sure you're protecting your joints, muscles, and overall well-being.

- **Warm up properly.** Prepping your muscles with dynamic stretches or light movement reduces the risk of injury. Think arm circles, hip openers, or a few bodyweight squats before strength training.

- **Cool down & stretch.** Taking 5–10 minutes to stretch post-workout helps your body recover, prevents stiffness, and improves flexibility.
- **Invest in proper footwear.** Shoes that support your arches and cushion your feet make all the difference—especially for walking, running, or strength training.
- **Listen to your body.** If something feels off, modify your movements and don't push through pain.

✦ **HOT TIP:** Joint pain? Swap high-impact workouts for low-impact options like swimming, cycling, or Pilates. You'll still get all the benefits without unnecessary strain.

Menopause is not the time to ignore injuries or overdo it. The right approach keeps you strong, resilient, and moving pain-free for years to come.

Step 6: Track Progress & Stay Motivated

Seeing your progress fuels motivation and keeps you consistent. Tracking doesn't have to be complicated—just find a method that works for you and stick with it.

- **Fitness Journal** – Write down workouts, set goals, and track consistency. Seeing your progress on paper makes it real.
- **Digital Calendars** – Block off workout times. Treat them like important meetings you can't cancel—because that's what they are.
- **Fitness Apps** – Try MyFitnessPal, Strava, or Apple Health to monitor workouts, calories burned, and progress.
- **Accountability Check-Ins** – Share wins with a friend, a trainer, or an online fitness group. A little external motivation goes a long way.

✦ **HOT TIP:** Track how you *feel*, not just the numbers. Did you have more energy? Sleep better? Feel stronger? Progress is about how movement improves your daily life, not simply calories burned or reps performed.

Consistency is where the magic happens. Even if progress feels slow, every step counts. Every minute you spend moving makes a difference. Keep showing up, and the results will follow.

3.3 MINDFUL EATING: LISTENING TO YOUR BODY'S SIGNALS

You've built a strong foundation with nutrient-dense foods and movement, but *how* you eat is just as important as *what* you eat. Mindful eating isn't about restrictions or rigid rules. It's about tuning in to your body's natural hunger and fullness cues, so eating becomes an act of nourishment, not habit, impulse, or a way to fill boredom.

During menopause, when your body feels like it's constantly shifting, this practice becomes even more powerful. Your metabolism, digestion, and cravings change, and learning to listen to your body's signals can help you feel more balanced, satisfied, and in control.

Eat with Awareness: Slow Down & Savor

Have you ever finished a meal and barely remembered eating it? That's the opposite of mindful eating.

Instead of rushing through meals on autopilot, mindful eating encourages you to slow down, engage your senses, and truly *experience* your food. When you savor each bite, notice the flavors and textures, and allow your body time to register fullness, you naturally eat in a way that supports digestion, energy levels, and satisfaction.

Focus on small, intentional shifts that transform the way you fuel your body.

Make Mindful Eating a Habit

Like any new practice, mindful eating takes time to develop. Start small—pick one meal a day where you remove distractions and fully engage with your food. Reflect on how you feel after meals and notice how tuning in affects your energy and digestion.

◆ **Your Challenge:** At your next meal, put your phone away, take a deep breath before eating, and savor each bite. What do you notice?

How to Start: Put your fork down between bites. This simple habit forces you to slow down. Chew thoroughly—digestion begins in your mouth, and slowing down helps your body absorb nutrients better. Breathe between bites. This resets your nervous system, helping you feel calm and connected to your meal.

✦ **HOT TIP:** Try the *first bite test*. Before diving into your next meal, take one bite and pause. Close your eyes and focus on the taste, texture, and sensation. This small act helps train your brain to enjoy food more fully and recognize when you're actually satisfied.

Recognizing Hunger vs. Emotional Eating

Sometimes we eat because we're truly hungry. Other times, it's because we're bored, stressed, or emotional. Menopause can heighten these emotional cravings, making it easy to reach for food as comfort rather than true nourishment.

The next time you reach for a snack, ask yourself:

- **Am I physically hungry?** (Stomach growling, low energy, poor focus?)
- **Am I thirsty?** (Dehydration can mimic hunger.)
- **Am I eating for distraction or comfort?** (Stress, boredom, or emotions?)

Instead, try this:

If it's physical hunger: Eat a balanced meal with protein, fiber, and healthy fats.

If it's emotional eating: Try one of these quick alternatives:

- **Take a 5-minute movement break**—walk, stretch, or step outside.
- **Drink a glass of water**—don't let dehydration trick you.
- **Engage your brain**—journal, knit, or do a small task to shift focus.
- **Call or text a friend**—sometimes, connection is what you really need.

By identifying *why* you're reaching for food, you build healthier coping mechanisms that don't rely on snacks to fill the void.

Eliminate Distractions & Be Present

We live in a world full of distractions—endless to-do lists, screens, and multitasking pull us away from our meals. But studies show that eating while distracted can lead to consuming **25% more calories** because your brain isn't registering fullness properly.

Creating a mindful eating environment requires only small adjustments. Turn off screens. Set aside your phone, TV, or laptop during meals. Sit down at a table. Avoid eating on the go or while standing in the kitchen. Create a mealtime ritual. Light a candle, play soft music, or simply take a deep breath before eating. Always have a glass of water with your meal. The more present you are at meals, the more satisfied and in tune with your body you'll feel.

Mindful Eating Benefits: Better Digestion & Blood Sugar Balance

Beyond the mental shift, mindful eating has physical benefits, too. Chewing thoroughly supports digestion, reduces bloating, and improves nutrient absorption. Eating slowly helps stabilize blood sugar, preventing energy crashes and cravings. And when you take time to enjoy food, you naturally eat the right amount —leaving you feeling satisfied rather than overly full.

3.4 SUPERFOODS FOR MENOPAUSE: WHAT TO ADD TO YOUR DIET

The term *superfoods* gets thrown around a lot, but what does it actually mean for menopause? These foods provide targeted benefits, from **balancing hormones** to **supporting brain health** and **reducing inflammation**. By incorporating more of them into your meals, you're actively working with your body's changing needs.

I first started paying attention to superfoods when I noticed my energy dipping and brain fog creeping in. I didn't want to rely on caffeine or quick fixes, so I started experimenting with small changes—adding flaxseeds to my oatmeal, throwing berries into my smoothies, and sipping turmeric tea in the evening. The difference was real. And the effort? Minimal.

Berries: The Ultimate Skin & Brain Boost

Blueberries, raspberries, and strawberries are loaded with antioxidants that protect against cellular damage, keeping your skin radiant and your brain sharp. Oxidative stress increases during menopause, which can accelerate aging and memory decline. Berries help fight inflammation, support cognitive function, and may even reduce the risk of heart disease.

Adding berries into your diet is effortless. Toss a handful into yogurt, oatmeal, or salads for an easy nutrient boost. Keep a bag of frozen berries in your freezer for quick smoothies or a refreshing snack. The best part? They satisfy a sweet craving without spiking your blood sugar.

✦ **HOT TIP:** The darker the berry, the higher the antioxidant content. Blackberries and blueberries pack the most powerful punch!

Nuts & Seeds: Small but Mighty

When it comes to healthy fats, brain function, and hormone balance, nuts and seeds are some of the best foods you can eat. I used to think of them as just snack foods, but now they're a staple in my daily meals.

Almonds are rich in vitamin E, which supports skin health and protects against cognitive decline. Walnuts are packed with omega-3s, which are anti-inflammatory and great for brain function. And then there are flaxseeds and chia seeds—two tiny but mighty sources of fiber and phytoestrogens that help balance hormones and improve digestion.

For an easy boost, sprinkle chia seeds into smoothies, oatmeal, or yogurt. Stir ground flaxseeds into soups or dressings (they need to be ground for your body to absorb their nutrients).

Snack on a handful of walnuts or almonds in the afternoon to keep your energy steady.

Flaxseeds: Nature's Hormone Balancer

One of the most fascinating things I learned about menopause nutrition is how flaxseeds contain plant-based estrogens that mimic estrogen in the body. Since menopause causes estrogen levels to decline, incorporating phytoestrogens may help regulate hormones naturally.

I started adding a tablespoon of flaxseeds to my morning oatmeal, and not only did my digestion improve, but I noticed fewer energy crashes throughout the day.

Want to try it? Mix ground flaxseeds into yogurt, smoothies, or even baked goods. They add a mild, nutty flavor and an incredible nutritional boost.

Turmeric: The Anti-Inflammatory Powerhouse

If I had to pick one superfood that's made a noticeable difference in how I feel, it's turmeric. This bright yellow spice contains curcumin, a compound that's been shown to reduce joint pain, fight inflammation, and support overall wellness.

I started incorporating turmeric into my diet when I noticed more stiffness in my joints, and now it's a daily ritual. Whether in a warming golden milk latte, sprinkled into scrambled eggs, or stirred into a soup, it's an easy, delicious way to reduce inflammation naturally.

✦ **HOT TIP:** Always pair turmeric with **black pepper**—it boosts absorption by up to 2,000%!

Bringing Superfoods to Your Plate

Superfoods work best when they're a seamless part of your routine rather than something you feel like you *have* to eat. I found that by making small swaps—choosing walnuts over croutons in salads, adding flaxseeds to dressings, and blending turmeric into my tea—these powerhouse foods became second nature.

Here are some simple ways to add them into your daily routine:

- **Superfood Smoothie** – Blend kale, mixed berries, flaxseeds, and almond milk for a refreshing, nutrient-packed start to your day.
- **Overnight Oats** – Soak oats with chia seeds, walnuts, blueberries, and cinnamon in almond milk for an easy, balanced breakfast.
- **Golden Turmeric Soup** – A blend of carrots, ginger, turmeric, and coconut milk makes for a nourishing, anti-inflammatory meal.

The Truth About Superfoods: No Magic Bullet

It's easy to get caught up in the hype around superfoods, but the reality is they aren't a magic cure-all. They work best as part of a balanced diet that includes lean proteins, whole grains, and plenty of colorful vegetables. The key is variety and moderation—not overloading on one food while neglecting others.

◆ **Your Challenge:** Try adding two superfoods to your meals this week and see how you feel! Whether it's flaxseeds in your smoothie or turmeric in your soup, small changes add up to big benefits.

3.5 HYDRATION AND HEALTH: THE IMPORTANCE OF WATER

Imagine your body as a finely tuned machine, with water as the essential lubricant keeping everything running smoothly. During menopause, hydration isn't just about quenching thirst. It's about regulating body temperature, keeping energy steady, and combating dryness from the inside out.

Hydration & Hot Flashes: Your Body's Built-In Cooling System

Ever noticed that hot flashes seem more intense when you're dehydrated? That's because water plays a direct role in your body's ability to regulate temperature. When you're properly hydrated, your internal cooling system works efficiently, helping to lessen the severity and frequency of heat surges.

Beyond keeping you cool, hydration is essential for your skin. As estrogen levels decline, your body's ability to retain moisture drops, leaving skin drier and less elastic. Drinking enough water supports a healthy glow, helps reduce itchiness and irritation, and strengthens your skin barrier. While beauty is a bonus, the goal is comfort and resilience.

Water also affects energy. Many people don't realize that sluggishness, brain fog, and even irritability can stem from dehydration. If you wake up feeling groggy, reaching for a glass of water before your morning coffee can help kickstart digestion and provide an instant energy boost.

✦ **HOT TIP:** Every morning drink a full glass of water before anything else. It rehydrates your body after sleep, helps flush out toxins, and can make a noticeable difference in how you feel.

How Much Water Do You Really Need?

The "8 glasses a day" rule is a good starting point, but hydration needs vary based on activity level, diet, and climate. A general rule of thumb is to aim for at least half your body weight in ounces—for example, if you weigh 150 lbs, aim for 75 ounces of water daily.

Your body will also tell you when it's running low. Signs of dehydration include dark urine, fatigue, dizziness, headaches, dry mouth, and bloating. If any of these sound familiar, it may be time to increase your water intake.

If hitting your hydration goal feels overwhelming, start small. Keeping a water bottle nearby, setting a reminder, or simply making water part of your routine—like drinking a glass before meals—can make it effortless.

Make Hydration Enjoyable

If plain water feels boring, there are plenty of ways to get creative:

- **Infused water** – Try fresh lemon, cucumber, berries, or mint to add natural flavor.
- **Herbal teas** – Caffeine-free blends like hibiscus, peppermint, or chamomile provide hydration with extra health benefits.
- **Electrolyte boosts** – Coconut water, electrolyte drops, or a pinch of Himalayan salt can help replenish minerals lost through sweat.

Personally, I love mixing Smith Teas green tea with peppermint tea and a splash of unsweet vanilla almond milk—it's a refreshing, antioxidant-packed way to hydrate while giving me a little boost of energy in the afternoon.

The Sneaky Effects of Dehydration

When you don't get enough hydration, everything slows down—your mind, digestion, and even your mood.

- **Brain fog & fatigue** – Dehydration makes it harder to focus and drains energy levels.
- **Mood swings & headaches** – Even mild dehydration can lead to irritability and tension headaches.
- **Digestive discomfort** – Low water intake can slow digestion, leading to bloating and constipation.

Before reaching for caffeine or a sugary snack, try a glass of water first. Many times, dehydration is the culprit behind mid-afternoon sluggishness.

Final Takeaway: Hydration Is Self-Care

Menopause comes with enough challenges—don't let dehydration make it harder. Small, simple hydration habits can have a huge impact on energy, skin, digestion, and mood.

◈ **Your Challenge:** Track your daily water intake for a week. If you're falling short, try adding one new hydration habit—whether it's a morning glass of water, a fun infused recipe, or a hydration app. After a few days, see how you feel!

3.6 ALCOHOL AND CAFFEINE: FRIENDS OR FOES?

Imagine a cozy evening, a glass of wine in hand, the perfect way to unwind after a long day. But as you sip, an unwelcome warmth creeps up, your skin flushes, and suddenly, a hot flash takes center stage. Alcohol, while a familiar companion, can exacerbate menopause symptoms like hot flashes, night sweats, and restless sleep. What once felt like a relaxing indulgence might now leave you tossing and turning, sweating through the sheets, or waking up feeling foggy.

Caffeine presents its own set of challenges. That morning coffee or afternoon latte may be non-negotiable, but its stimulating effects can worsen anxiety, trigger palpitations, and disrupt sleep. You might need that extra cup to power through the afternoon slump, but later, you're staring at the ceiling at midnight, wondering why sleep won't come. Menopause heightens your body's sensitivity to both alcohol and caffeine, making it more important than ever to pay attention to their effects.

Alcohol & Menopause: A Delicate Balance

I used to love beer. A crisp, cold pint at the end of a long day? Perfection. But when my doctor ran a blood test and flagged new food sensitivities—wheat, corn, soy, and peanuts—beer was suddenly off the table. This was more than a minor inconvenience. It was a major shift in my social life and habits. What had once been my go-to drink was now a surefire way to trigger inflammation, bloating, and discomfort.

So, I pivoted. I moved to vodka sodas, thinking they'd be the perfect replacement. And while I do love a good vodka soda, I quickly learned that sometimes they hit me a lot harder than expected. One drink could leave me feeling completely fine, while another would sneak up on me with a surprising intensity. Eventually, I found that hard seltzers, while not my first love, were more predictable. Their standardized alcohol content meant fewer surprises, and they became my safe bet for social occasions.

This experience reinforced something menopause was already teaching me: what worked before doesn't always work now, and that's okay. Our bodies change, our tolerances shift, and paying attention to what fuels us—versus what drains us—makes all the difference.

Alcohol & Menopause: The New Rules of the Game

With lower estrogen levels and a slower metabolism, drinks hit harder, linger longer, and often come with side effects that make them less fun than they used to be.

"Alcohol is like a pause button on your health goals. One drink a week? No big deal. Three to four drinks a week? You're pressing pause on progress multiple times." — Emily Howell, WCS

What Alcohol Can Do During Menopause:

- **Trigger hot flashes & night sweats** – Alcohol dilates blood vessels, amplifying heat surges.
- **Disrupt sleep cycles** – Even if it helps you relax during the early evening, alcohol interferes with REM sleep, leading to restless nights and groggy mornings.
- **Affect mood stability** – That evening drink might take the edge off initially, but it can lead to heightened anxiety or irritability later.
- **Increase belly fat storage** – With a slower metabolism, alcohol is more easily stored as fat, especially around the midsection.

Finding a Balance That Works for You

Instead of an all-or-nothing approach, menopause calls for adjusting, experimenting, and listening to your body. I had to navigate this shift myself, moving away from beer and figuring out what made me feel good rather than just sticking to old habits or completely cutting certain things out of my life.

- **Pay attention to how different drinks affect you.** Some people handle wine better, while others (like me) find spirits more tolerable.
- **Stick to one drink per day (or less)** and see how you feel. Notice if certain drinks impact your sleep, mood, or hot flashes more than others.
- **Experiment with alternatives.** Lower-alcohol wines, dry-farmed wines, or spirits with fewer additives may be easier on your system.
- **Hydration is key.** Alcohol dehydrates you, and dehydration worsens menopause symptoms. Alternating drinks with water can help.

✦ **HOT TIP:** If you're feeling off after drinking, check in with yourself. Was it the type of alcohol? The amount? The timing? Keeping a simple note in your phone after social outings can reveal patterns you might not otherwise notice.

Caffeine: The Love Affair with Limits

My morning coffee? Still a non-negotiable. But that second cup? The afternoon iced coffee? The pre-workout boost? That's where things got tricky.

Caffeine used to be a simple pleasure—drink it, feel energized, get things done. Boom, end of story. But menopause makes its effects feel stronger and more unpredictable. Some days, coffee still works like magic. Other days, it leaves me jittery, anxious, or staring at the ceiling at 2 a.m.

Caffeine isn't inherently bad. In fact, it has some great perks:

- **Packed with antioxidants** that support brain health and reduce inflammation.
- **May lower the risk of cognitive decline** and even protect against Alzheimer's.
- **Can boost focus and metabolism** when consumed in moderation.

But Here's the Catch...

Caffeine sensitivity increases during menopause, meaning that what used to be a harmless pick-me-up can now feel like an instant ticket to anxiety town. If you're experiencing heart palpitations, sleep disruptions, or an afternoon energy crash, it might be time to reassess your intake.

How to Keep Caffeine in Your Life Without the Side Effects:

- **Limit caffeine after noon** to prevent sleep disruption.
- **Switch to lower-caffeine options** like matcha, half-caff coffee, or mushroom coffee blends.
- **Pair caffeine with food** (especially protein or healthy fats) to slow absorption and avoid energy crashes.
- **Listen to your body.** If you feel wired, jittery, or anxious, scale back and see if symptoms improve.

✧ **HOT TIP:** If you love coffee but want to cut back, try blending decaf with regular coffee for a half-caff option. It still gives you a little boost and the flavor, but without the extreme highs and lows.

Final Takeaway: Balance Over Perfection

I didn't stop drinking altogether when I realized beer no longer worked for me—I adapted. The same goes for caffeine. Menopause isn't about cutting out everything you love. It's about adjusting so you can keep feeling your best. If something is making you feel off, experiment with small changes and see what works.

◈ **Your Challenge:** Pay attention to how alcohol and caffeine affect your body this week. Notice if certain drinks impact your sleep, mood, or hot flashes. Try making one small adjustment—like switching from beer to a lower-alcohol option or swapping an afternoon coffee for herbal tea—and see if it makes a difference.

Chapter Wrap

Menopause changes how your body responds to food, movement, and yes—alcohol. But instead of seeing it as a loss, think of it as intel. Every shift is a clue. Every choice is a chance to feel more like yourself. And now that you've got the basics of fueling your body, it's time to dig into the tools that help bring balance—from herbs and acupuncture to cutting-edge therapies.

Next up? Let's talk about what treatments—from supplements to HRT—can actually help.

Nourishing Your Body: Nutrition and Lifestyle

KEY Takeaways

1. Prioritize 25–30g fiber and 80–100g protein daily.
2. Strength training preserves metabolism and bone density.
3. Alcohol intolerance and new food sensitivities are common.

HOT TIPs

- Build meals: protein plus fiber plus healthy fats.
- 2-3x/week strength train for energy & metabolism.
- Limit alcohol to one drink max or opt for mocktails.

ACTION ITEMS

- [ ] Post the Eat Me infographic on your fridge.
- [ ] Buy The One Life Planner (and thank me later).
- [ ] Add one new high-fiber food to your daily diet.
- [ ] Track alcohol intake and notice body response shifts.

Resources

- Web: NutritionFacts.org
- Book: The Menopause Reset by Dr. Mindy Pelz
- Instagram: @dr_mosconi
- Podcast: The Happy Menopause by Jackie Lynch

NEXT UP — *Get ready for Chapter 4: exploring herbs, supplements, adaptogens, acupuncture, and the new science behind holistic relief.*

4

STARTING POINTS: NATURAL, ALTERNATIVE, AND EMERGING THERAPIES

Menopause isn't a one-path journey—and it sure isn't one treatment fits all. While hormones often steal the spotlight, there's a whole world of powerful therapies that support your body, mind, and spirit without relying on hormone replacement therapy (HRT).

This chapter is your guide to the wider menu. We'll dig into acupuncture, acupressure, herbal medicine, adaptogens, supplements, and emerging therapies like cognitive behavioral therapy for menopause (CBT-M), hypnosis, and new non-hormonal pharmaceuticals. You'll also get a glimpse into promising peptide therapies.

Whether you're starting here, layering these tools alongside HRT, or simply looking for extra support, you deserve to know what's available. You'll find ideas backed by research, grounded in real-world experience, and served up with a healthy dose of "take what you need, leave what you don't."

Before You Dive In

Menopause relief isn't about choosing "natural" *or* "medical." It's about finding the right combination for *you*.

Some people build a strong foundation with acupuncture and adaptogens. Others turn to emerging pharmaceuticals or cognitive therapy to shift symptoms without touching hormones. Many use these therapies as powerful add-ons to hormone treatment.

Here's the bottom line:

- Alternative and complementary therapies can offer real symptom relief, especially for stress, sleep, mood, and hot flashes.
- These options can be used alone or layered with HRT for even better results.
- You deserve a toolkit that's as flexible and adaptive as you are.

This chapter is about expanding your choices. Let's find the tools that help you thrive.

4.1 ACUPUNCTURE AND ACUPRESSURE: EASTERN RELIEF FOR WESTERN SYMPTOMS

Imagine lying in a dimly lit room, soft music playing in the background, and feeling a sense of calm wash over you as tiny needles are placed along your body. This is acupuncture, a practice rooted in Eastern medicine that's been used for thousands of years. For some, it feels like tapping into an ancient form of magic; for others, it's simply a moment of quiet relief in an otherwise chaotic life.

Acupuncture and acupressure are based on the concept of **Qi** (pronounced "chi"), which is believed to be the life force or energy that flows through the body along pathways called **meridians**. According to this philosophy, when these pathways are blocked or out of balance, it can lead to physical and emotional issues.

Acupuncture involves inserting thin needles into specific points along these meridians to restore balance and harmony, potentially alleviating symptoms like hot flashes, insomnia, and mood swings. Acupressure follows the same principle but uses finger pressure instead of needles—making it a needle-free alternative for those who might be squeamish.

So... Does It Work?

Here's where things get interesting: **some studies show that acupuncture works, while others suggest it's more of a placebo effect**. For example, the Acupuncture in Menopause (AIM) Study found that women who received acupuncture reported fewer and less intense hot flashes, better sleep quality, and improved mood. Other research has linked acupuncture with reduced anxiety and increased overall well-being.

But not all studies have been as conclusive. Some researchers suggest that the benefits of acupuncture may be largely due to the placebo effect—the idea that the act of receiving treatment itself creates a psychological shift that helps relieve symptoms. But does it really matter if the relief comes from the placebo effect or the treatment itself? If it works for you, it works.

This is where the "choose your own adventure" nature of menopause treatment comes into play. If you've tried everything else and acupuncture is something you're curious about (or have benefited from in the past), it's absolutely worth exploring. Even if the science isn't 100% settled, relief is relief—and that's what matters.

My Experience

I've used acupuncture many times throughout my life. Do I know if it actually changed anything on a physiological level? Nope. But did I dig it? Absolutely. There's something about the ritual of it—the quiet, the deep breathing, the sensation of energy moving through my body—that left me feeling calmer and more grounded. And when you're riding the rollercoaster of menopause, that feeling alone can be worth it.

The biggest challenge for me isn't whether acupuncture works —it's finding the time to make it happen. There are only so many hours in the day, and when I'm choosing how to manage my symptoms, I have to think about which treatments give me the most bang for my buck, both in time and money. That's why I think of acupuncture, acupressure, and even massage as **more than just physical treatments**. They're also about the focus and intention behind taking care of yourself. And that, in itself, is valuable.

What to Expect

If you're considering acupuncture or acupressure, the first step is to talk to your healthcare provider. While acupuncture is generally safe, it's important to make sure it won't interfere with any medical conditions or medications you're taking.

From there, it's about finding a licensed, experienced practitioner who understands menopausal symptoms. A typical acupuncture session lasts about **30 to 60 minutes**. The needles are so thin that you'll barely feel them (or not at all), and many people find the experience deeply relaxing. Acupressure can be more accessible since you can learn to do it yourself at home or work with a massage therapist or practitioner for guidance.

Consistency matters. Relief from acupuncture and acupressure tends to build over time, so if you're considering it, plan for a series of sessions rather than expecting overnight results. You might feel some improvement after the first visit, but most benefits come after **4 to 6 sessions**.

Are There Risks?

Acupuncture and acupressure are generally safe when performed by trained professionals. Some people might experience mild bruising or soreness at the needle sites, but this usually passes quickly. It's essential to ensure that your acupuncturist uses sterile, single-use needles to prevent any risk of infection.

Certain conditions—like bleeding disorders or severe skin sensitivity—might require caution or even rule out acupuncture altogether. That's why it's crucial to have an open conversation with both your doctor and your practitioner before starting treatment.

Why It Might Be Worth It

For some women, acupuncture and acupressure feel life-changing. For others, they're just an expensive nap. But even if the relief is tied to the placebo effect, is that really a problem? If it makes you feel better and helps you cope with the physical and emotional chaos of menopause, that's a win.

What I've learned is that menopause is not a linear journey—it's a highly personal one. Acupuncture and acupressure may or may not be the solution for you, but they're part of the wide range of options you have to create your own version of symptom relief. If you're curious, try it. If it works for you, fantastic. If it doesn't, that's okay too. This is your menopause adventure—there's no wrong way to find your path through it.

4.2 HERBAL REMEDIES: AN EVIDENCE-BASED APPROACH

When menopause hits, many women instinctively reach for nature's medicine cabinet. Herbal remedies have been used for centuries to manage hormonal shifts, and for good reason—plants have long been powerful allies for supporting health and balance. In fact, for many women, herbs are the first stop on their menopause journey. They offer a gentler, more familiar starting point before exploring medical treatments like HRT.

Herbs like **black cohosh** and **red clover** have been studied for their potential effects on hot flashes, mood swings, and bone health. While the scientific evidence is mixed, many women swear by these remedies—and traditional wisdom often holds weight even when modern research struggles to keep up. The key is to approach herbal remedies with both respect and awareness. Just because something is natural doesn't mean it's risk-free, and not all herbs play nicely with other treatments (including HRT).

Why Herbs Are a Popular First Step

Herbs have an undeniable appeal. They're accessible, familiar, and have fewer side effects than many pharmaceuticals. For women who are hesitant about starting HRT—or whose symptoms aren't yet severe enough to consider medication—herbs offer a natural way to test the waters. The ritual of brewing a cup of red clover tea or taking a tincture of black cohosh can also feel grounding and empowering—a signal that you're actively caring for your body.

I've turned to herbal remedies myself at different points in my life. Black cohosh helped me when my hot flashes were starting to spike. Did it fix everything? No. But it took the edge off and gave me enough relief to sleep through the night, which was a gift in itself. For me, the biggest benefit of using herbs, acupuncture, and massage is the sense of focus and intention it creates around my health. Even when the impact is subtle, it feels good to take action.

What the Research Says

Black cohosh is one of the most well-studied herbs for menopause, especially for reducing hot flashes and improving sleep. Some studies suggest it may work by interacting with serotonin receptors, which could explain its effects on temperature regulation and mood. But the research isn't entirely consistent—some trials show clear improvements, while others haven't found a significant difference. That said, for many women, the personal results speak louder than the data.

Red clover is rich in **isoflavones**—plant compounds that mimic estrogen in the body. Some studies suggest that red clover can help with bone health and mild hot flashes, but others have been less conclusive. Still, the fact that it works for some women is reason enough to explore it. Traditional wisdom often leads where science is still catching up.

It's important to know that most herbs—aside from black cohosh—haven't been studied extensively for their long-term effectiveness in treating menopause symptoms or side effects. That doesn't mean they aren't helpful, but it does mean you should proceed with some caution. If you're planning to use herbal remedies over a longer period, keep the conversation going with your doctor to make sure your approach stays safe and effective.

Other popular menopause-supporting herbs include:

- **Dong quai** – Often used in traditional Chinese medicine to balance hormones and improve circulation.
- **Evening primrose oil** – May help with breast tenderness and mood swings, though research is limited.
- **St. John's Wort** – Known for its mood-boosting properties, but it can interact with medications (including antidepressants and birth control).

Herbs won't necessarily work for everyone, but they've provided meaningful relief for many women. The key is listening to your body and being open to experimenting.

Combining Herbs with HRT—Proceed with Caution

If you're considering herbal remedies, talk to your healthcare provider first—especially if you're also using (or considering) HRT. Some herbs interact with hormones and medications in ways that can either enhance or reduce their effects. For example, red clover's estrogen-like properties could conflict with certain types of HRT, and St. John's Wort can affect how your body metabolizes medications.

✧ **HOT TIP:** Herbal remedies are most effective when they're high-quality. Look for third-party tested products that list the plant's Latin name, the part of the plant used, and the dosage. Organic products and those with minimal fillers are often a safer bet.

This is why working with a menopause-savvy doctor, naturopath, or herbalist is so important. They can help you navigate the best combinations of herbs and medical treatments (if needed) without risking adverse interactions.

Why It's Worth Exploring

Herbs are not a second-tier option or a stepping stone to "real" treatment—they're a legitimate and meaningful part of many women's menopause journeys. If they work for you, embrace that. If they don't, keep experimenting until you find the right mix.

Menopause is a choose-your-own-adventure experience, and herbal remedies are just one of the paths you can explore. If they give you relief, that's a win. If they don't, you've learned something about your body and can adjust your approach. The key is to stay open, stay curious, and build a strategy that works for your unique body and life.

4.3 ADAPTOGENS: FOCUSING ON STRESS MANAGEMENT

When your hormones are doing the cha-cha and your stress response is in overdrive, you might hear someone mention **adaptogens**. These are herbs and natural substances that help your body better handle stress. Not eliminate it entirely (we wish), but *adapt*—hence the name. During menopause, when estrogen dips and cortisol spikes, that extra support can make a meaningful difference.

Adaptogens aren't magic pills, but they can be helpful tools—especially when combined with other healthy habits. I recently added **rhodiola** to my morning routine before workouts, and I'm loving the gentle boost. It helps me feel more energized and focused without feeling overstimulated, which is exactly the kind of support I need on days when motivation is dragging. That's the sweet spot with adaptogens: subtle, supportive shifts that help your body function a little more smoothly when everything feels like too much.

So, what are adaptogens?

Adaptogens are herbs and fungi that help regulate your body's stress response, especially by supporting the **HPA axis** (the connection between your brain and adrenal glands). This system can get thrown off during menopause, leading to fatigue, anxiety, sleep disruptions, and general "I'm losing it" vibes. Adaptogens don't flood your system with hormones or push your body in an aggressive direction. They're more like trusted sidekicks that help your body stay balanced through chaos.

They've been used in traditional medicine systems for centuries, and modern research is starting to catch up. While the studies are still emerging, there's promising evidence that certain adaptogens may support **energy, focus, mood, sleep, and resilience to stress**—all of which are pretty clutch during this hormonal rollercoaster.

A Quick Guide to Common Adaptogens

There are dozens of adaptogens out there, but these six are among the most widely used during menopause—and for good reason. Each one has its own personality and area of focus, so it's worth exploring what aligns with your current needs. This chart offers a quick breakdown of what they're best for, when to take them, and who might benefit most.

🌿 Use this as a starting point—not a prescription.

Adaptogen	Best For	When to Take	Try This First If...
Ashwagandha	Stress, anxiety, sleep	Evening	You're wired but tired and need help calming down
Rhodiola	Fatigue, brain fog, low motivation	Morning	You need a lift without a jittery crash
Maca	Energy, mood, stamina, libido	Morning or mid-day	You're feeling flat, foggy, or disconnected
Reishi	Sleep, immune support, calm	Evening	You're tired but restless and getting sick often
Schisandra	Resilience, mood, mental clarity	Morning	You feel depleted and cranky
Holy Basil	Mood swings, mild	Anytime	You want a gentle calm

✦ **HOT TIP:** Most people start with one adaptogen and give it 2–4 weeks to work. You can build from there, but don't pile on too many at once. Your body doesn't need to be overwhelmed—it's already doing enough.

Where Adaptogens Fit in Your Treatment Plan

Adaptogens can be a great starting point if you're not ready for HRT or want to explore natural support first. They also pair well with hormone therapy, especially if you're looking to improve **energy, mood, and stress tolerance** without adding more prescriptions to the mix.

They work best as part of a whole-body approach: solid sleep, nourishing food, joyful movement, meaningful connections, and regular check-ins with a provider who supports your goals. Like everything else in menopause, it's all about layering the right tools to support *your* unique system.

A quick word of caution: adaptogens can interact with medications (especially blood pressure or thyroid meds), so talk to your provider before adding them in. Ideally, you're working with someone who respects both Eastern and Western perspectives —and, more importantly, someone who *listens*.

How They Feel (and How They Don't)

Don't expect a dramatic overnight change. Most adaptogens work gently and gradually. The benefits often show up in quiet ways: a little more stamina at work, fewer doom spirals at 2 a.m., less snapping at your partner for breathing too loud. But if you start feeling off—too flat, too revved up, too tired—pay attention. That's your signal to adjust the dose, take a break, or try a different one.

Potential Side Effects and Things to Watch For

While adaptogens are generally considered safe, they're not without quirks. Pay attention to how your body reacts, especially when you're just starting out.

- **Mild GI issues** – Nausea or diarrhea can happen, especially with higher doses.
- **Hormonal effects** – Maca and ginseng may have mild hormonal activity.
- **Overstimulation** – Rhodiola, eleuthero, and ginseng can feel too buzzy if taken in large amounts.
- **Allergic reactions** – Rare, but worth noting.
- **Blood pressure shifts** – Ginseng and schisandra can raise or lower blood pressure, depending on the person.

As always, check with a provider—especially if you're taking medications, have high blood pressure, or are managing hormone-sensitive conditions.

Adaptogens + Menopause: FAQs

Q: Can I combine adaptogens with HRT?

A: Yes. Many people use adaptogens alongside hormone therapy to support energy, mood, and stress. Just make sure your provider is in the loop.

Q: How long do they take to work?

A: Some adaptogens (like rhodiola or ashwagandha) may start helping within a few days, but most take 2–4 weeks to notice full effects.

Q: Are they safe for everyone?

A: Generally, yes—but people with autoimmune issues, high blood pressure, or hormone-sensitive cancers should use caution and talk to a doc first.

Q: What's best for hot flashes?

A: American ginseng and schisandra have shown promise. Maca may help balance hormones and reduce night sweats too.

Q: Can they affect sleep?

A: Yep. Ashwagandha and reishi are great for winding down. Rhodiola and ginseng? Save those for the morning.

Q: Can I combine more than one?

A: Sure—but go slow and pair them strategically.

- **Morning:** Rhodiola, ginseng, cordyceps (energy + focus)
- **Evening:** Ashwagandha, reishi, schisandra (calm + sleep)

Q: Are adaptogens regulated by the FDA?

A: Nope. They're classified as supplements, so regulation is minimal. Look for third-party tested brands for safety and quality.

Q: Can they help with menopause weight gain?

A: Indirectly, yes. By lowering cortisol and supporting energy and mood, they may reduce stress eating and help you get moving again.

Q: What's the best adaptogen for low libido?

A: Maca and Asian ginseng are popular choices. Ashwagandha may also help by reducing stress and gently boosting testosterone.

Q: Do they affect thyroid function?

A: Some do. Ashwagandha and maca may increase thyroid hormone levels, so check with your provider if you're on thyroid meds or have hyperthyroidism.

A Gentle Invitation

If stress, fatigue, or brain fog are dragging you down, and you're not quite ready for bigger interventions—or you're already doing a lot and want to round out your plan—adaptogens might be worth exploring. Start with one. Give it time. Check in with yourself and your care team. And remember: you don't need to *do all the things* to feel better. You just need the right ones for you.

4.4 THE ROLE OF SUPPLEMENTS: FINDING THE RIGHT BOOST

If herbal remedies are nature's medicine cabinet, supplements are like a personal toolkit—offering targeted support for the physical and emotional shifts of menopause. For many women, supplements are an easy and practical starting point. They're accessible, relatively affordable, and don't require a prescription, which makes them an appealing way to address some of the most common menopause symptoms.

Supplements can't replace a balanced diet, medical treatment, or lifestyle changes, but they can fill in the gaps and give your body an extra boost where it needs it most. And during menopause, there are some very real gaps to fill. The decline in estrogen levels that comes with menopause affects everything from bone density to mood to cardiovascular health. That's where supplements can step in, offering targeted support to help you feel more balanced and resilient.

Why Supplements Matter

Some of the most well-supported supplements for menopause focus on **bone health, heart health, and energy levels**—areas that are particularly vulnerable during this stage of life.

- **Calcium** and **vitamin D** top the list for bone health. As estrogen declines, so does bone density, increasing the risk of osteoporosis. Calcium provides the building blocks for strong bones, while vitamin D helps your body absorb that calcium. Without enough of both, even a calcium-rich diet might not be enough to prevent bone loss.
- **Omega-3 fatty acids** are well-known for their heart health benefits, but they also reduce inflammation and

may help improve mood and cognitive function. Studies have linked omega-3s to a reduced risk of cardiovascular disease—a growing concern as estrogen's protective effects wane.
- **Vitamin B12** plays a critical role in energy production, mood regulation, and cognitive function. It becomes especially important as you age, since your body's ability to absorb B12 naturally decreases over time. If you're feeling unusually tired or foggy, low B12 could be part of the problem.
- **Magnesium** often flies under the radar, but it's essential for muscle function, sleep quality, and mood. Some women find that magnesium helps with night cramps, restless legs, and even anxiety.

These aren't just nice-to-haves—they're fundamental to keeping your body strong and balanced as you navigate menopause.

That said, not every supplement has the same level of scientific backing. Some menopause-targeted products—like those promising to "restore hormonal balance" or "eliminate hot flashes overnight"—are more marketing than science. That's why it's important to approach supplements with a mix of curiosity and caution.

My Experience

I've leaned on supplements at different times throughout my menopause journey. When I started feeling more fatigued than usual, a B12 supplement helped me feel sharper and more energized. Magnesium became part of my nightly routine when I realized it helped me sleep better and reduced those annoying nighttime muscle cramps. And while I try to get most of my calcium from food, adding a supplement gave me peace of mind that I was supporting my bone health long-term.

Do I think supplements fix everything? No. But I absolutely think they help fill in the cracks. And sometimes, when you're deep in the thick of menopause, even a small edge can make a meaningful difference.

Finding the Right Fit

The supplement aisle can be overwhelming. Slick packaging and bold claims can make it hard to know what's worth your money. Here's how to cut through the noise:

✦ **HOT TIP:** Look for third-party testing certifications, like NSF International or ConsumerLab. These organizations test for purity and potency, ensuring that what's listed on the label is actually in the bottle.

Be wary of supplements with fillers, artificial dyes, or excessive additives. Supplements should list the plant or nutrient's scientific name, the source, and the dosage. If the label is vague or the ingredient list is suspiciously long, that's a red flag.

You'll also want to consider how the supplement fits into your overall health plan:

- Are you already getting enough of the nutrient from your diet?
- Do you have any underlying health conditions that could interact with the supplement?
- Are you taking medications that might conflict with certain nutrients?
- What are you hoping this supplement will help with? And how will you know it is working?

This is where talking to a menopause-savvy doctor or nutritionist matters. They can help you identify where you have gaps and where you're better off relying on whole foods or lifestyle changes instead.

The Bottom Line

Supplements are practical, accessible, and often effective. If you're curious about them, try them. If they help, keep them. If they don't, move on. The goal isn't to follow a set formula—it's to build a personalized strategy that helps you feel your best.

Menopause is a layered experience, and supplements are one piece of the puzzle. They might not be the whole solution, but they can absolutely be part of it. And when you find that right mix of support—whether it's through food, supplements, lifestyle changes, or all of the above—that's when things really start to click.

4.5 NEW AND INNOVATIVE THERAPIES: EXPANDING THE TREATMENT LANDSCAPE

Menopause is a time of change, but it's also a period ripe with innovation. New therapies—and a few long-standing ones finally getting the attention they deserve—are expanding the options for managing symptoms like hot flashes, mood swings, and sleep disturbances.

Hormone replacement therapy (HRT) remains a cornerstone of menopause treatment, but today, non-hormonal and targeted pharmaceutical options are offering new paths to relief, especially for those who can't or prefer not to use hormones.

The key takeaway? If traditional treatments haven't worked for you (or you've been hesitant to try them), there's a growing list of scientifically-backed alternatives that are worth exploring. Let's take a closer look at some of the most promising options.

Non-Hormonal Pharmaceutical Options

Non-hormonal medications are gaining traction as legitimate, effective treatments for menopausal symptoms. While they were originally designed for other conditions, research has shown that they can provide meaningful relief for menopause-related issues.

- **Fezolinetant** (sold as **Veozah**) – FDA-approved Veozah targets **neurokinin receptors** in the brain, which are involved in regulating body temperature. By modulating these receptors, Veozah reduces the frequency and severity of hot flashes. Unlike HRT, it works independently of estrogen levels, making it a game-changer for women who can't or don't want to use hormone-based treatments.
- **SSRIs and SNRIs** – Certain antidepressants, including paroxetine (Brisdelle), venlafaxine (Effexor), and desvenlafaxine (Pristiq), have been shown to reduce hot flashes and improve mood stability. Unlike hormone-based treatments, these medications work on serotonin and norepinephrine levels in the brain, helping to regulate body temperature and emotional balance. Bridelle has FDA approval and is the lowest dose of an SSRI, so less side effects (hint hint: weight gain) than many other antidepressants.
- **Gabapentin** – Originally developed for nerve pain and seizures, gabapentin has been shown to reduce the severity and frequency of hot flashes. Its effectiveness seems to stem from its ability to modulate how the brain regulates body temperature.
- **Clonidine** – This blood pressure medication has also been found to help with hot flashes, although it's less

commonly used due to potential side effects like dizziness and dry mouth.

These non-hormonal options are particularly valuable for women with a history of breast cancer or other conditions that make HRT unsuitable. They offer a way to manage symptoms without affecting estrogen levels or increasing certain health risks.

Alternative and Mind-Body Therapies

Beyond pharmaceuticals and supplements, a growing number of mind-body and alternative therapies are helping women navigate menopause with more ease. While these approaches might not eliminate symptoms completely, they can improve overall well-being and resilience.

- **Cognitive Behavioral Therapy with Mindfulness (CBT-M)** – CBT-M has been shown to reduce the emotional intensity of hot flashes and improve sleep quality. By teaching coping strategies and helping to reframe thoughts around menopause, CBT-M can improve emotional stability and resilience.
- **Hypnosis** - Research suggests that hypnosis can significantly reduce the frequency and severity of hot flashes, often after just a few sessions. Many women continue to experience lasting benefits over time. There are even FDA-cleared hypnosis apps available to support ongoing practice at home.
- **Yoga and Tai Chi** – These mind-body practices help reduce stress, improve flexibility, and promote relaxation. Studies have shown that they may reduce the frequency and intensity of hot flashes and improve mood stability.

- **Acupuncture** – While research on acupuncture is mixed, many women report feeling more balanced and relaxed after regular sessions. The stimulation of specific points on the body may help regulate body temperature and improve mood.

What's Not Ready for Prime Time

While the therapies above are backed by clinical research, others are still in the newer or experimental stages. Take peptide therapy, for example—it's been a buzz in wellness circles, but most of the existing research is limited to animal studies or small trials.

- **BPC-157** – A synthetic peptide that may promote tissue repair and reduce inflammation. Currently, human studies are limited, and it's not FDA-approved for menopausal symptoms.
- **PT-141** – A peptide being explored for sexual function, but most research is in early stages. Potential side effects, including nausea and flushing, have raised concerns about its safety profile.

Experimental therapies like these may hold promise down the road, but they aren't yet ready to be considered alongside FDA-approved treatments. For now, they're more curiosity than solution.

The Expanding Landscape of Menopause Treatment

What's clear is that the range of options for managing menopause is broader than ever before. Traditional HRT remains an effective and well-researched choice for many women, but the rise of non-hormonal pharmaceuticals and targeted therapies means that relief is no longer limited to estrogen.

If your current approach isn't giving you the results you need—or if you've been hesitant to try hormone therapy—there are now more options than ever to explore. From neurokinin inhibitors to natural adaptogens and mind-body practices, menopause treatment is no longer a one-size-fits-all proposition.

The most empowering part of this shift? You get to choose. Whether you find relief through medication, herbs, lifestyle changes, or a mix of all three, the goal is to create a menopause experience that works for your body and your life.

- **For mild symptoms or early exploration**: Start with herbs, adaptogens, and lifestyle shifts.
- **For moderate to severe symptoms**: HRT is safe and effective for most, especially if you're under 60 or within 10 years of menopause.
- **For those who can't or don't want HRT**: Non-hormonal meds, CBT-M, acupuncture, and more may offer meaningful relief.

4.6 WRAPPING UP: BUILDING YOUR TOOLKIT, LAYER BY LAYER

The therapies we've explored in this chapter—acupuncture, acupressure, herbal remedies, adaptogens, CBT-M, supplements, and emerging treatments—offer real and meaningful ways to support your body through menopause. For many women, especially those in early perimenopause, these options are a fantastic place to start. If something resonates with you, go for it. You deserve the chance to try therapies that feel right for your body, your philosophy of care, and your life.

That said, it's important to understand the scope of what natural and alternative therapies can offer. Many of these approaches are excellent at treating symptoms one by one—improving sleep, easing anxiety, calming hot flashes, or boosting energy. But when you start needing support across multiple systems at once, HRT often becomes the more powerful, foundational tool. Instead of chasing symptoms individually, HRT can address the root hormonal shifts that are creating the domino effect in the first place.

We'll dive much deeper into HRT in the next chapter, but I want you to start noticing something now, especially if you're experiencing symptoms yourself or seeing them in friends.

Once you hit your mid-thirties and beyond, many traditional Western medicine doctors still treat perimenopausal symptoms separately rather than connecting the dots. If you walk into an appointment complaining of insomnia, low libido, anxiety, and joint pain, you might leave with a sleeping pill, an antidepressant, and some vague suggestions about exercise—without anyone ever mentioning that you're likely in perimenopause.

You have to be on alert for that.

If you're seeing signs like irregular periods, increased anxiety, sleep issues, temperature sensitivity, or brain fog, it's time to start thinking about menopause-specific care. You deserve providers who are willing to step back and see the bigger picture, not just treat symptoms piecemeal.

None of this is about pushing you toward one "right" way to treat menopause. If herbs, acupuncture, adaptogens, and lifestyle changes are giving you what you need, that's beautiful. Stick with it, build on it, and layer your support however it works best for you.

But it's also important to know the limits—and the possibilities. As Dr. Kaley Bourgeois explains:

"You can take as much soy, red clover, and black cohosh as you want, and they might help a little with symptoms like sleep or hot flashes. But none of them will give you the hormone levels your body actually needs if you're trying to restore energy, maintain metabolism, and protect bone density."

There's a place for natural therapies.

There's a place for mind-body support.

And there's a place for hormone therapy.

The key is knowing when to explore, when to build, and when to level up your support.

In the next chapter, we'll step fully into the world of hormone replacement therapy—clearing up the myths, understanding how it works, and showing why, for many of us, HRT isn't a backup plan. It's the real foundation for thriving in this next chapter of life.

Starting Points: Natural, Alternative, and Emerging Therapies

KEY Takeaways

1. Relief matters more than "natural" or pharmaceutical.
2. Layer treatments like herbs + lifestyle + targeted support.
3. Third-party testing is vital when choosing supplements or herbs.

HOT TIPs

- Adaptogens often take 3–6 weeks to show full effect.
- Look for NSF, USP, or ConsumerLab seals on supplements.
- Layer 1 natural therapy (like Reishi) + 1 lifestyle shift (like CBT-M).

ACTION ITEMS

- [ ] Explore 2 non-HRT treatments for one of your symptoms.
- [ ] Ask your provider about trying CBT-M, acupuncture, or herbal support.
- [ ] Commit to one 10-minute daily practice: deep breathing, stretching, or guided meditation.
- [ ] Review one supplement you take on Labdoor, Examine.com, or ConsumerLab for safety, dosing, and quality.

✦ Resources ✦

- Web: menopause.org Hormone Therapy
- Book: The Hormone Cure by Dr. Sara Gottfried
- Instagram: @dr.avivaromm
- Podcast: On Health with Aviva Romm

NEXT UP

Chapter 5 takes a fearless look at hormone therapy: what's safe, what's outdated, and how to build an HRT plan that fits your specific health and hormone profile.

5

HORMONE REPLACEMENT THERAPY: THE GOLD STANDARD FOR MENOPAUSE CARE

When it comes to reclaiming your well-being during menopause, hormone replacement therapy often stands out for a reason. For most people, it's not just effective—it's life-changing.

In this chapter, we're breaking through outdated fears and myths. You'll learn why modern HRT is safe for the vast majority of women, especially when started within 10 years of menopause. We'll explore the differences between systemic and localized therapy, plant-derived versus synthetic hormones, and what "bioidentical" really means (hint: it's not just about being "natural"). We'll also dive into compounded hormones—and when they're helpful or risky.

This isn't about pushing you into a decision. It's about giving you clear, science-backed information so you can make the choice that feels right for your body, your values, and your future.

Before You Dive In

There's a lot of noise out there about hormone therapy—and some of it is wrong.

Here's what you need to know before we get started:

- HRT is the most effective treatment for hot flashes, night sweats, bone loss, and many other menopause symptoms.
- Starting HRT early (within 10 years of menopause) provides the greatest benefits with the least risk.
- FDA-approved "Bioidentical" hormones are safe and effective; compounded hormones require extra caution and oversight.
- Localized (vaginal) estrogen therapy can dramatically improve quality of life with minimal systemic risk.
- You are the expert on your own comfort and goals—and you deserve care that supports both.

If you've been curious, confused, or even a little scared about HRT, you're in the right place. This chapter is about real information, real empowerment, and real options.

5.1 INTRO TO HORMONE REPLACEMENT THERAPY

As you progress through perimenopause and your hormone levels really start tanking, menopause can feel like a storm you can't control, and you're searching for a lifeline. You've tried every natural remedy in the book, but the hot flashes are relentless, like a mischievous imp that keeps appearing at the most inconvenient times. Your nights are filled with tossing and turning, and you find yourself longing for a solution that offers real relief.

This is where **hormone replacement therapy** enters the conversation—a topic shrouded in both promise and apprehension. HRT isn't just a buzzword; it's a medically approved approach that replaces the hormones your body is no longer producing in sufficient amounts, particularly **estrogen** and **progesterone**. For many women, HRT is the difference between sleepless nights and finally waking up rested, between emotional rollercoasters and feeling balanced again.

One of the first things we have to tackle is the decades-long misinformation surrounding the safety of HRT.

5.2 THE BENEFITS AND RISKS (AND THE TRUTH ABOUT *THAT* WHI STUDY)

The benefits of HRT can be life-changing. Imagine cutting the frequency and intensity of your hot flashes in half—or better yet, sleeping through the night without waking up drenched in sweat. HRT can also improve mood stability and prevent bone loss, which reduces the risk of fractures as you age.

Christina Cameli, CNM, puts it this way:

> "I love that I've learned enough about hormone therapy to feel really safe using it. After nearly two decades of prescribing contraceptive hormones, making the transition to menopausal hormones was natural. It's not for everyone, and it won't solve every problem, but for mood changes, hot flashes, night sweats, and insomnia, it can make a huge difference."

But it's not a miracle cure, and it's not without risks. The **Women's Health Initiative (WHI) study** falsely raised alarms about increased risks of breast cancer, stroke, and blood clots with systemic HRT. This 2002 study triggered widespread fear and caused many women and doctors to avoid HRT altogether. Because menopause is talked about so little, many women approach menopause with these fears in the back of their mind, a kind of, "I don't know the specifics, but I know hormone replacement therapy will give me cancer" sentiment.

The thing you need to know is that the WHI study was flawed: the participants were older—many of them already past menopause—the subject groups were not randomized, and they were using synthetic hormones. **Subsequent research and reanalysis have shown that the initial findings were misinterpreted and overstated**. The increased breast cancer risk was linked to a specific combination of estrogen and progestin (a synthetic progesterone), not bioidentical hormones. For women who begin HRT **before the age of 60** or within **10 years of menopause**, the overall health benefits tend to outweigh the risks. For instance, transdermal estrogen (like a patch) appears to carry a lower risk of blood clots compared to oral estrogen.

The message here isn't that HRT is risk-free—it's that the risks need to be seen in context. And for many women, the benefits—particularly for relief of hot flashes, mood regulation, night sweats, and bone health—can be significant.

Dr. Bourgeois points out that, for the majority of women, HRT is a safe and effective option—except for rare cases, such as with a personal or family history of certain types of cancer or clotting disorders. She recommends having your family medical history readily available when you discuss HRT.

5.3 SYSTEMIC VS. LOCAL HRT

HRT comes in two primary forms: **systemic** and **local**.

- **Systemic HRT** is designed to enter your bloodstream and affect your entire body. It can be delivered through oral pills, skin patches, gels, a vagina ring or injections. Systemic HRT is typically used to treat a broad range of menopause symptoms—hot flashes, night sweats, mood swings, and more.
- **Local HRT** targets specific areas, like the vaginal region, and is often used to treat dryness, discomfort during intercourse, or urinary issues. Since local treatments don't circulate through the whole body, they tend to have fewer systemic side effects.

5.4 BIOIDENTICAL HORMONES: WHAT THEY ARE—AND WHAT THEY AREN'T

Let's start with the basics: **bioidentical hormones** are hormones that are chemically identical to the ones your body naturally produces.

Molecule-for-molecule, they match. When you use an FDA-approved estradiol patch, for example, your body can't tell the difference between that estrogen and the estrogen you made yourself at age 25.

That's the real benefit of bioidentical hormones.

It's not about where they come from—it's about whether your body recognizes the structure. A bioidentical hormone fits into your body's hormone receptors like a key fitting perfectly into a lock. No jiggling. No forcing. Just a smooth, natural connection.

Sometimes people hear the word "bioidentical" and assume it automatically means "natural."

Not exactly. Let's break that down—because understanding this difference could save you a lot of confusion (and a lot of money).

Let's dig a little deeper.

5.5 NATURAL VS SYNTHETIC: CUTTING THROUGH THE CONFUSION

If you spend even five minutes online, you'll find influencers tossing around the words "natural" and "synthetic" like they're obvious, black-and-white categories.

In reality? It's a lot messier—and marketing plays a huge role in shaping what we believe.

> "Right now, menopause conversations are dominated by people trying to sell you something—coaching programs, supplements, expensive hormone therapy. The ads make it seem like your body is betraying you and only they have the fix. That messaging is so gross to me."
>
> — CHRISTINA CAMELLI, CNM

Christina puts it bluntly—and she's right. There's a lot of noise out there, and it can make it hard to tell what's real, what's helpful, and what's just hype. So let's get clear on what these terms actually mean when it comes to hormone therapy

Here's the deal:

✦ **Plant-derived bioidentical hormones include:**

- **Estradiol:** Estrogen made from yams or soy, chemically identical to human estrogen.
- **Micronized progesterone:** Progesterone from yams, again a perfect molecular match to human progesterone.

Sounds natural, right? And in a sense, it is. These hormones start out in plants, but they still have to be **synthesized in a lab** to be transformed into something your body can use.

The final product is a carefully engineered hormone that happens to be made from plant ingredients. No matter what the label says, you are not rubbing wild yams on your skin and magically balancing your hormones.

On the other hand:

✦ **Synthetic and animal-derived hormones include:**

- **Premarin:** Estrogen sourced from pregnant mare urine (the name literally stands for "PREgnant MARes' urINe").
- **Ethinyl estradiol:** A synthetic estrogen found in many birth control pills.
- **Medroxyprogesterone acetate (MPA):** A chemically altered progestin used in older HRT options.

These hormones are incredibly important for many people and still widely used. They don't perfectly match human hormones, but they're close enough to provide real benefits for managing menopause symptoms when needed.

That said, **bioidentical hormones offer the advantage of a perfect molecular match.** Your body recognizes them as its own, often leading to smoother absorption and fewer surprises.

In short:

- "Natural" is mostly a marketing word.
- Plant-derived hormones are still lab-synthesized.
- **Structure—not source—is what matters most to your body.**

Now that you know the difference, let's talk about another source of confusion: **how your hormones are made and delivered.**

5.6 FDA-APPROVED VS COMPOUNDED BIOIDENTICAL HORMONES

Even within the world of bioidentical hormones, not all options are equally safe—or equally reliable.

Here's where the fork in the road shows up:

✦ **FDA-Approved Bioidentical Hormones:**

- These include pills, patches, gels, creams, vaginal rings, and suppositories.
- They're rigorously tested for safety, potency, and consistency.
- When you pick up an FDA-approved product, you get standardized dosing and a detailed list of known risks and side effects.

✦ **Compounded Bioidentical Hormones:**

- These are custom-mixed formulas created by compounding pharmacies—often tailored into creams, lozenges, or gels.
- They aren't subject to FDA testing or oversight.
- Dosing can vary from batch to batch, and risk information may be incomplete or missing.

The appeal of compounded hormones makes sense:

If you need a specific dose that isn't available off-the-shelf, or if you're allergic to an ingredient like the peanut oil used in some progesterone capsules, a customized option can be life-changing.

As Christina Camelli, CNM, points out, compounded hormones are a valuable tool *when there's a real medical reason to customize*. But she also warns that the idea of compounded hormones being "more natural," "safer," or "better" is mostly marketing—not science.

And here's the critical safety issue:

When dosing isn't consistent—especially with progesterone—you run real risks.

If you're using estrogen without enough real protection for your uterus, you could increase your risk of endometrial cancer. Progesterone creams rubbed on your skin may sound gentle and natural, but they aren't reliably absorbed the way oral progesterone is—and your uterus needs reliable protection.

So how do you navigate this?

- If you need customization, work with a knowledgeable provider who understands menopause medicine—and a reputable pharmacy.
- If you don't have a specific reason to go compounded, **FDA-approved bioidentical hormones are the safest, most predictable choice.** And typically most affordable.

Quick Takeaway

- **Bioidentical** means your body sees the hormone as its own—not that it came straight from nature.
- **Natural vs synthetic** is mostly marketing noise. What matters is the structure—and how well it fits your body's locks and keys.
- **FDA-approved vs compounded** isn't about snobbery—it's about safety, consistency, and trust in what you're putting in your body.

The bottom line?

You deserve treatments that work *with* your body, not just ones that sound good on a label. Choose wisely. Trust yourself.

5.7 MY EXPERIENCE WITH HRT

My own experience with HRT was a journey of discovery. I've never been much of a pill popper—vitamins and herbs were more my style. But when menopause hit and hot flashes, night sweats, and insomnia started wreaking havoc on my life, I knew I needed to explore my options. My doctor and I worked together and landed on a plan that included progesterone, magnesium, and environmental changes—things like lowering the bedroom temperature, using essential oils, and creating a calming nighttime routine.

A few months later, my estrogen levels had tanked, so we added biweekly estradiol patches.

Recently, Dr. Bourgeois pointed out something funny about the real-life messiness of starting HRT that I didn't even realize. She said, *"You were one of my most inconsistent patients. Took a year to get you to use your hormones consistently. But once you did—you were like, these are wonderful!"*

And she's right. Since I've gotten consistent with it, I've loved the results. Who would've thought that giving up beer and bread would be easier than committing to taking my hormones regularly?

Dr Bourgeois also emphasizes that if the first treatment plan doesn't work, it's important not to give up. You can always try different forms of hormones and adjust the doses until you find what works for you. Even after that, keep in mind that your needs will continue to evolve as you progress through menopause, and your treatments will likely need to evolve with them.

5.8 THE BOTTOM LINE

The goal here isn't to convince you that HRT or bioidentical hormones are the answer. It's to encourage you to approach your options with an **open mind**. There's no single "right" path through menopause. Whether you choose HRT, bioidentical hormones, or other therapies, the important thing is that you feel informed, supported, and empowered to make the decision that's right for you.

For me, adding progesterone and estradiol patches was a game-changer. It helped me sleep better, eased my mood swings, and reduced my hot flashes. But it was part of a broader plan that included lifestyle changes and magnesium. The goal isn't just to survive menopause—it's to thrive through it. Bioidentical hormones can be part of that equation, but they aren't the whole solution.

"Gen X has crushed this assignment! Broken the silence, lifted each other up, and insisted on clear information and science"

— CHRISTINA CAMELI, CNM

Hormone Replacement Therapy: The Gold Standard

KEY Takeaways

1. HRT is safest before 60 and within 10 years of menopause.
2. FDA-approved bioidenticals are reliable and widely available.
3. Personalization is key—form, dose, and timing all matter.

HOT TIPs

◆ Know your HRT: pills, patches, creams, rings.

◆ Be wary of "natural" miracle cures for menopause.

◆ Discuss FDA-approved bioidenticals with your provider.

ACTION ITEMS

☐ Research the difference between systemic and local HRT options.

☐ Download the NAMS HRT decision chart or bring a printed copy to your appointment.

☐ Create a list of HRT questions to discuss with your healthcare provider.

☐ Track any changes after starting HRT to fine-tune your plan.

✳ Resources ✳

- Web: North American Menopause Society (NAMS)
- Book: Estrogen Matters by Dr. Avrum Bluming and Carol Tavris
- Instagram: @dr_naomipotter
- Podcast: Let's Talk Menopause

NEXT UP — *In Chapter 6, we dive into building your personal dream team — from menopause-literate doctors to coaches to the right kinds of community support to help you thrive.*

6

BUILDING A SUPPORTIVE HEALTH TEAM

6.1 FINDING THE RIGHT DOCTOR: ADVOCACY AND COMMUNICATION TIPS

Picture this: You're standing tall, determined to tackle this next chapter of life with grit and grace. You're navigating the maze of menopause, and suddenly, it hits you: your healthcare team, the ones guiding you through this journey, feels more like a hindrance than a help. I've been there. I've stood at that crossroads, questioning whether the advice I'm getting is truly best for me. It's a moment of clarity. The status quo simply won't do.

"If your doctor dismisses your symptoms or tells you to just do NutriSystem instead of addressing perimenopause—find a new doctor. Your provider should care about this being a unique phase of your life."

— CHRISTINA CAMELI, CNM

You deserve a healthcare provider who understands menopause and respects your journey. Finding the right doctor is like finding a partner in your health—a collaboration built on trust, expertise, and mutual respect. It's about assembling a team that sees you as the unique individual you are, facing a transformative time in your life.

To your doctor's credit, Dr. Bourgeois notes most doctors get very little menopause training in school and those who are knowledgeable often pursue post-grad education by choice.

> "Most of what I learned about hormone therapy and menopause care was through continued education after I started practicing. The base training on it is very poor."
>
> — DR BOURGEOIS

Hear me loud and clear: this is not the time to stick with a doctor because you've been with them forever, they seem to have your best interest at heart, or you're worried about hurting their feelings. This chapter of your life is too important for that. You owe it to yourself to work with someone who is specifically trained and deeply experienced in navigating menopause—someone who truly gets it and knows how to help you feel like yourself again.

The first step is finding a provider who understands menopause care. Specialization matters—someone with a background in women's health or endocrinology will have the expertise to guide you through the hormonal shifts and health changes that come with this stage of life.

The Menopause Society offers a certification called the Menopause Society Certified Practitioner (MSCP), which ensures that a provider has specialized training in menopause care. Checking credentials and patient reviews can help you gauge whether a provider is a good fit. Trust your instincts—if you feel dismissed or unheard, it's probably not the right match.

Building a strong doctor-patient relationship goes beyond credentials. You need to feel comfortable talking about your symptoms and health goals without fear of being brushed off or judged. A good provider listens, validates your concerns, and works with you to create a plan that feels right for your body and lifestyle. Mutual respect matters—if your doctor values your input and engages with your questions, you'll feel more confident about following their recommendations.

Preparation helps, especially when navigating complex symptoms or treatments. Jot down your symptoms and questions ahead of your appointment so you don't forget anything important. Being clear and direct about what you need—whether that's medication, lifestyle changes, or simply more information—makes it easier for your doctor to offer the right support.

Dr. Bourgeois explains that she needs to hear "all the weird shit", even the stuff you're not sure is hormone related. Why? . Because it all helps paint a fuller picture. The more your care team knows, the better they can connect the dots and address the real root of what is going on. Nothing is too small, too strange, or too unrelated to mention. Speak up. It matters.

And if you feel nervous, bringing a trusted friend or family member to the appointment can help you feel grounded and ensure you remember key details afterward.

Sometimes, even when you've done everything right, you might still feel like you're not getting the care you need. That's when seeking a second opinion becomes invaluable. If two providers offer conflicting advice, take time to evaluate their reasoning and how each recommendation aligns with your health goals. You know your body best—trust yourself to make the right call.

I vividly remember the frustration of feeling unheard when my then-doctor suggested a diet plan that felt more like a throwback to a bygone era than a genuine solution. That moment was a turning point. I realized I had two choices: accept the status quo or take charge. I chose the latter, reaching out to my former trainer, Emily Howell, who recommended Dr. Bourgeois.

The wait for that first appointment was agonizing, but also transformative. I had time to clarify what I truly wanted for my health. When I finally met Dr. B, the experience was unlike any I'd had before. She listened—*really listened*—and together, we crafted a personalized plan that addressed my unique needs.

The takeaway? Finding the right doctor—and being willing to part with the wrong one—changed everything for me. While not everyone needs a naturopath, everyone deserves a care team that listens and respects their concerns. Whether your team includes a doctor, trainer, midwife, therapist, or more, the right support can help you take control of your menopause experience and step into your power. It's how I became a menopause unicorn, and it's a path you can follow too.

6.2 THE MENOPAUSE COACH: A GUIDE TO PROFESSIONAL SUPPORT

Imagine having someone in your corner, guiding you through the ups and downs of menopause like a seasoned tour guide in uncharted territory. A menopause coach offers just that—personalized support tailored to your unique experience. They provide accountability and motivation, helping you stay on track with your health goals.

A good menopause coach can be the catalyst that turns confusion into clarity, offering insights into lifestyle adjustments and stress management strategies tailored to ease your symptoms. With their help, you can navigate this phase with confidence, knowing you have a knowledgeable ally by your side.

What a Menopause Coach Can Do

A menopause coach focuses on practical, day-to-day support. While a doctor might prescribe medication or order tests, a coach helps you integrate that guidance into your life in a sustainable way. They can help you:

- Fine-tune your nutrition and develop a meal plan rich in phytoestrogens to help manage hot flashes and mood swings.
- Create an exercise routine to support bone density, muscle tone, and overall health.
- Offer stress-reducing techniques like mindfulness practices and breathwork to stabilize mood and improve sleep.
- Provide emotional support and a judgment-free space to process the emotional toll of menopause.

A menopause coach helps you see the big picture—how sleep, stress, diet, and movement all work together to influence your symptoms. They also help you problem-solve when setbacks arise, ensuring you feel supported rather than discouraged.

Finding the Right Menopause Coach

Like any professional relationship, the fit matters. A coach's qualifications and philosophy should align with your needs and values. Look for someone with formal training or certifications in menopause support. The Menopause Society and other reputable organizations offer certification programs, ensuring that coaches have evidence-based knowledge.

Recommendations from healthcare providers can be helpful, as they often know who's credible in the field. It's also valuable to have an initial conversation with a potential coach to assess their approach. Do they listen? Are they open to blending different strategies, such as combining lifestyle changes with medication if needed? You should feel comfortable being honest about your symptoms and health goals without fear of judgment. Trust is essential. You need to feel like you're working with someone who gets you.

Weighing the Investment

Working with a menopause coach is an investment, both financially and emotionally. Coaching rates vary, with some offering packages that include a set number of sessions or ongoing monthly support. While the cost can seem daunting, consider the long-term benefits: improved health, better symptom management, and potentially fewer medical expenses down the line. A coach can help you avoid the trial-and-error cycle that often comes with menopause care, steering you toward solutions that actually work.

The right coach will empower you to take control of your health. That sense of confidence and clarity is invaluable.

6.3 EMPOWERING CONVERSATIONS: SPEAKING UP ABOUT SYMPTOMS

Imagine walking into your doctor's office, determined to finally get some answers about the symptoms that have been hijacking your life. You know that articulating these symptoms clearly is the key to receiving the care you deserve.

Start by describing your symptoms with precision. Instead of saying, "I'm tired all the time," try, "I feel fatigued every afternoon around 3 p.m., despite getting seven hours of sleep." This kind of specificity helps your healthcare provider understand the nuances of your experience.

Using symptom trackers can be incredibly beneficial. They serve as visual aids, offering concrete data that can pinpoint patterns or triggers you might not notice in daily life. Whether it's a digital app or a handwritten journal, tracking your symptoms can illuminate connections and provide a comprehensive view of your health. This approach not only aids your doctor but also empowers you by giving you control over your narrative.

Fun fact: when I told my doctor that I was consistently getting up at 7 a.m. and hitting the gym, but it still felt *extra rough*, she paused and really listened. That simple detail—along with other symptoms I'd tracked—led her to suggest Wellbutrin. She explained that it could help with my mood, motivation, energy, and even weight management.

That conversation changed things for me. And it happened because I spoke up—and got specific..

I'm sharing this because we have to break down the stigma. Your treatment plan should work for *you*—and that starts with open, honest conversations.

Open discussions with family and friends can be a lifeline, offering emotional support when you need it most. Sharing your personal stories and struggles helps others understand what you're going through, fostering empathy and connection. It's not just about finding someone who will listen; it's about creating a network of understanding and support.

Encourage those around you to ask questions and express their feelings too. This mutual exchange can lead to deeper connections and a more supportive environment. Talking about menopause shouldn't be taboo. It's a natural phase of life, and discussing it openly can help dismantle the stigma that often surrounds it.

Sometimes, starting these conversations can feel daunting, especially if you're not used to speaking up about personal health issues. Practicing in safe environments can build your confidence. Whether it's role-playing with a friend or writing down what you want to say, rehearsing can ease anxiety and help you express yourself more clearly when the time comes.

Support groups, whether online or in-person, offer a platform to practice these conversations. They provide a space where you can share your experiences and gain feedback, helping you refine how you communicate your needs. These communities are invaluable, offering not only practice but also camaraderie and validation.

Advocacy in healthcare involves being an active participant in your health decisions. It's about understanding your rights and responsibilities and using this knowledge to make informed choices. Knowing what you're entitled to can empower you to push for the best care possible.

Patient advocacy resources are there to help you navigate the complexities of healthcare systems. They can guide you in understanding medical jargon, preparing for appointments, and ensuring your voice is heard. Being an advocate means standing up for yourself and ensuring that your health remains a priority, no matter the obstacles you face.

6.4 UNDERSTANDING HEALTHCARE OPTIONS: MAKING INFORMED CHOICES

Navigating healthcare options during menopause can feel like wandering through a vast and unfamiliar landscape. On one side is the conventional route with its specialists, prescriptions, and hormone therapies. On the other is the path of integrative and holistic care, offering alternatives like acupuncture, herbal remedies, and lifestyle changes. But the truth is, the right path isn't always obvious—and you don't have to choose just one.

Conventional medicine offers targeted relief. Gynecologists and endocrinologists are trained to address the hormonal shifts of menopause, providing treatments like HRT and prescription medications to ease symptoms like hot flashes and mood swings. For many women, HRT is life-changing, restoring balance and dramatically improving quality of life. But it's not the only option.

Some providers are trained to bridge the gap between conventional and holistic care. As a naturopath, Dr. Kaley Bourgeois offers a blended approach. She prescribed HRT and antidepressants but also helped me adjust my diet after identifying new food sensitivities, recommended vitamins to support hormone balance, and even suggested environmental changes like adjusting my sleep routine and using a fan.

Specialists like Christina Cameli—a certified midwife and menopause expert—also take this whole-person approach, combining medical knowledge with lifestyle guidance. Finding someone with this kind of broad training means you don't have to compartmentalize your care. You get a unified, tailored plan that addresses your whole experience.

Staying informed is your best ally. You don't need to become an expert, but understanding the science behind different treatments empowers you to have better conversations with your healthcare provider. Read clinical studies, ask your doctor about new research, and don't be afraid to challenge information that feels off. At the same time, real-world experience matters too. Forums, support groups, and even social media can offer insight from women navigating the same journey. Hearing what's worked—and what hasn't—for others can help you refine your own plan.

Personalized care is the foundation of good menopause management. Your needs will evolve over time, and what works now might need adjusting in six months or a year. That's why regular check-ins with your provider are essential. The goal isn't just to survive menopause—it's to thrive through it.

6.5 INSURANCE INSIGHTS: NAVIGATING COVERAGE AND COSTS

Navigating the world of health insurance can feel like deciphering a foreign language, especially when it comes to menopause care. Understanding what your insurance covers is crucial. Typically, health insurance plans provide coverage for consultations, treatments, and certain medications related to menopause. However, the specifics can vary widely depending on your policy.

It's important to carefully review the terms and conditions of your plan to know what is included and any limitations that might apply. Be aware of deductibles, co-pays, and out-of-pocket maximums, as these will affect your expenses. Some plans cover HRT, while others might not. Knowing these details in advance can save you from unexpected bills and ensure you're prepared to make informed decisions about your care.

Start with Your Healthcare Provider's Office

Your first step should be to speak with the billing or administrative staff at your healthcare provider's office. They often have direct experience with different insurance companies and can help you understand what's covered and what isn't. Many offices will even contact your insurance company on your behalf to confirm coverage before starting treatment. They can also advise you on which treatments are more likely to be approved or if you need a referral or pre-authorization.

When I was considering HRT, I wasn't sure if my plan covered it. The office staff at my doctor's office called my insurance company, confirmed the details, and verified coverage. If you're feeling overwhelmed, let them help—this is part of their job.

Maximizing Your Insurance Benefits

Maximizing your insurance benefits requires a strategic approach. Take advantage of preventive care services, which are often covered at no additional cost. Regular check-ups and screenings can help catch issues early and manage symptoms effectively, reducing the need for more extensive treatment later on. If you encounter a denied claim, don't hesitate to appeal.

- Gather all necessary documentation, including doctor's notes and lab results.
- Communicate clearly with your insurance provider and keep detailed records of all interactions (including dates, names, and outcomes).

- Many denied claims can be overturned with the right information—don't give up after the first rejection.

If you feel stuck, patient advocacy groups can help you navigate complex claims and denials.

Dealing with Coverage Limitations

Insurance coverage for menopause care can be inconsistent. Some plans cover HRT and antidepressants, while others may exclude them or limit coverage to certain types of medications. Alternative treatments like acupuncture, supplements, or therapy may not be covered at all. If you discover that a necessary treatment isn't covered, don't lose hope.

- **Ask about cash payment rates** – Some providers offer discounts for direct payments rather than going through insurance.
- **Explore supplementary coverage** – A secondary insurance policy or membership-based healthcare plan may offer better menopause-related coverage.
- **Seek assistance from insurance advocates** – Groups like the **Patient Advocate Foundation** (www.patientadvocate.org) can help negotiate with insurance companies and find solutions.

✣ **HOT TIP:** Denied claim? Appeal it. Many are overturned if you persist with documentation and clarity.

Managing Out-of-Pocket Expenses

Flexible Spending Accounts (FSAs) and Health Savings Accounts (HSAs) are valuable tools for managing healthcare costs. These accounts allow you to set aside pre-tax dollars for medical expenses, which can be used to cover co-pays, deductibles, and non-covered treatments.

- **FSAs** – Offered through most employer-sponsored plans; funds typically must be used within the calendar year.
- **HSAs** – Available for people with high-deductible health plans; funds roll over year to year and can grow with interest.

If you're still facing a large bill, don't hesitate to ask your provider about payment plans. Many healthcare offices are willing to work out a structured plan that allows you to pay over time rather than all at once.

Helpful Resources

If you need more help understanding your coverage or advocating for better care, these resources are a good place to start:

- **HealthCare.gov** – Official government site for health insurance options and coverage (www.healthcare.gov)
- **The Patient Advocate Foundation** – Helps patients resolve insurance coverage and payment disputes (www.patientadvocate.org)
- **The Menopause Society** – Offers guidance on menopause care and finding providers (www.menopause.org)
- **State Insurance Commissioners** – Each U.S. state has an insurance commissioner's office that can help you with coverage disputes or provider issues (find yours at www.naic.org)

6.6 BUILDING YOUR SUPPORT NETWORK: FAMILY, FRIENDS, AND PROFESSIONALS

Imagine standing at the center of a web of support, each strand a lifeline. During menopause, this network becomes your safety net, offering emotional, practical, and professional support. Family and friends play a crucial role, providing the understanding and empathy that only those close to you can offer. They see you at your best and your worst, and their support can make navigating this challenging time more manageable.

Open communication is vital. Share your needs and experiences with your loved ones to create a space where everyone feels comfortable expressing their feelings. Don't assume they know what you're going through—menopause is still a mystery to a lot of people. Let them know how they can support you, whether that's giving you space, helping with logistics (like covering the school run when you're wiped out), or just listening without judgment.

Setting boundaries is equally important. You deserve time and space to process changes at your own pace, so don't hesitate to protect your energy when you need to.

Professional guidance is another pillar of your network. Healthcare providers offer the expertise needed to manage the physical aspects of menopause, but don't overlook other professionals who can play a key role. Therapists provide emotional support, while nutritionists can help you adjust your diet to meet your changing needs. A menopause coach or specialized provider (like a naturopath or midwife) can help you bridge the gap between medical and holistic care. Combining these resources creates a whole-body support system that works together, with each member contributing their expertise to help you thrive.

But some of the most valuable connections come from talking to other people who are going through it too. Joining a support group—whether online or in person—creates a sense of solidarity that's hard to find elsewhere. Hearing that someone else is struggling with the same sleep issues or brain fog makes you feel less alone. You might pick up new coping strategies or just feel reassured that you're not imagining things.

You've already heard the story—me, center track, sweating through my shirt, declaring I was in menopause and handing out hot flash fans like Oprah. That moment cracked open the conversation—but what really changed me were the quiet ones that followed.

Skaters and audience members came up to me afterward, telling me their stories, asking questions, exhaling with relief. One of them mentioned her doctor had recommended Wellbutrin, but she wasn't sure if she should take it. When I told her I had—early on, to help with mood and motivation—her shoulders dropped. We're both "not depressed" people, but we shared a look that said, *This is harder than we expected, and that's okay.*

After 21 years leading Rose City Rollers, I know people trust me to shoot straight. So I've leaned into that trust—not as a menopause expert, but as someone who's in it and willing to talk. Those ripple effects? They matter. When we share—even the vulnerable stuff—we give others permission to do the same.

Whether you're an introvert or an ultra-extra extrovert like me, connection matters. Shared experiences, mutual curiosity, honest stories—this is how we build a culture where menopause isn't taboo, it's just another season of life we get through together.

So build your web. Bring together your people, your pros, your fellow travelers. Let them hold you up when you're tired and cheer you on when you find your spark again. This support network won't just carry you through—it'll help you rise.

Building a Supportive Health Team

KEY Takeaways

1. Most healthcare providers receive minimal menopause training.
2. You deserve individualized, respectful treatment options.
3. Support teams amplify success — build yours now!

HOT TIPs

- ◆ Treat finding a provider like hiring a contractor: interview.
- ◆ Bring symptom data and goals to appointments.
- ◆ Consider menopause coaching for personalized strategy and support.

ACTION ITEMS

- ☐ Find a menopause-certified provider — NAMS.org has a free directory.
- ☐ Bring your health history and symptom timeline to appointments.
- ☐ Join an online or local menopause support group.
- ☐ Research menopause coaches in your area.

✻ Resources ✻

- Web: menopause.org Find a Provider tool
- Book: What Fresh Hell Is This? by Heather Corinna
- Instagram: @letstalkmenopause
- Podcast: Women's Health Unplugged with Dr. Jordan Robertson

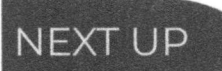

You've built your team — now it's time to rebuild emotional connections, reignite intimacy, and nurture relationships in Chapter 7

7

EMBRACING EMOTIONAL AND MENTAL WELLNESS

7.1 YOUR NEW TOOLKIT: PREPARING FOR YOUR EMOTIONAL AND MENTAL JOURNEY

Emotional wellness during menopause is about more than just managing symptoms. It's about finding balance and reclaiming your sense of self. The emotional shifts that come with menopause are the direct result of hormonal changes. As estrogen levels drop, the brain's regulation of mood, sleep, and even memory becomes disrupted. Cortisol—the body's primary stress hormone—often rises, making you feel more anxious, irritable, and emotionally unsteady.

Research has shown that practices that calm the nervous system —like mindfulness, meditation, and breathwork—can help reduce cortisol levels and improve emotional stability. But emotional wellness goes beyond calming techniques. Taking care of your mental health means building a foundation of resilience—learning to manage stress, nourish your emotional well-being, and embrace the changes your body is going through rather than resisting them.

That means developing a toolkit of strategies that work together:

- **Mindfulness and meditation** – Techniques to anchor yourself in the present and manage hormonal shifts with greater calm.
- **Self-care strategies** – Practical ways to nourish your body and mind, including sleep hygiene, stress management, and emotional boundaries.
- **Journaling** – How tracking your experience can reveal patterns and deepen self-awareness.
- **Letting go and embracing change** – Finding strength in transformation and rewriting the menopause narrative on your terms.

While we can't eliminate uncomfortable emotions, we can create space for them while giving ourselves the tools to move through them with clarity and confidence. This chapter will guide you in building that foundation.

7.2 MINDFULNESS AND MEDITATION FOR MENOPAUSE: FINDING YOUR INNER PEACE

Mindfulness and meditation train your brain to handle stress, improve focus, and create emotional balance. When hormonal changes leave you feeling emotionally volatile or mentally foggy, mindfulness helps you reset.

The strength of mindfulness lies in its simplicity. It's not about silencing your thoughts; it's about learning to observe them without judgment. Meditation deepens that skill, creating space for stillness and focus when emotions feel overwhelming.

Why Mindfulness and Meditation Matter During Menopause

Hormonal shifts can trigger intense emotional reactions—sometimes faster than you can process them. Regular mindfulness practice helps calm your nervous system, reducing the stress response before it spirals. Research shows that mindfulness techniques like mindful breathing or guided meditation can lower cortisol levels, improve sleep quality, and even reduce the frequency of hot flashes (*Journal of Clinical Psychology*, 2018).

Another powerful benefit? Mindfulness has been shown to improve sexual function in menopausal women. A 2020 study published in *Menopause* found that mindfulness increased body awareness and reduced anxiety around physical changes, making it easier to reconnect with your body during intimacy.

Getting Started with Meditation and Mindfulness

You don't need hours of silence or a special room to get started. Simple techniques like these can quickly become part of your routine:

- **Guided Imagery** – Close your eyes and imagine a calming scene—a forest, a beach, or any place that brings you peace. As you immerse yourself in the imagery, your body will naturally relax.
- **Loving-Kindness Meditation** – Sit comfortably and silently repeat phrases like, *"May I be happy, may I be healthy, may I be at peace."* This practice is especially helpful on days when irritability or anxiety feels overpowering.
- **Body Scan** – Lie down or sit comfortably. Starting at your toes, mentally scan your body, noticing sensations without judgment. Release tension as you move upward.

This simple practice helps you tune into your body's needs without frustration.
- **Mindful Breathing** – Sit quietly, focus on your breath, and gently bring your attention back whenever your mind wanders. This simple practice is highly effective for easing anxiety and promoting calm.

✦ **HOT TIP:** Practicing mindful breathing for as little as **5 minutes a day** has been shown to improve emotional control and reduce cortisol spikes. Try linking it to an existing habit—like your morning coffee or brushing your teeth—to make it stick.

Overcoming Common Meditation Challenges

Starting a mindfulness practice can feel frustrating at first, especially if your mind is racing. Here's how to handle common roadblocks:

- **Racing thoughts** – Don't try to empty your mind; instead, practice noticing your thoughts without attaching to them. Imagine they're passing clouds—acknowledge them, then let them drift by.
- **Restlessness** – If sitting still is hard, try a walking meditation. Focus on the rhythm of your steps and the sensations in your feet as they connect with the ground.
- **Lack of time** – Short sessions are just as effective. Even two minutes of intentional breathing can create a noticeable shift.

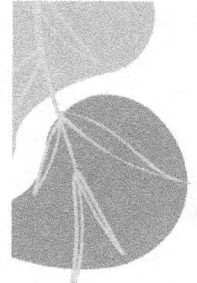

MEDITATION: CALMNESS

Lie down in a comfortable position and close your eyes. Take a deep inhale, hold for 3 seconds, then deeply exhale. Repeat this breathing pattern 5 times, then continue breathing normally.

While focusing on your breath, relax your whole body. Feel total relaxation and the total absence of daily distractions, obligations, and tasks. Feel all those aspects of your life falling off you, away from you, and disappearing. Feel how insignificant those daily duties are.

Feel this moment right here, right now.

Once you have totally released all external obligations, imagine yourself as the sky. Feel yourself as that vast space. Feel the broadness, the wideness, and the endless expansion.

Now, feel the changes you go through as the sky. Feel the clouds coming and going. Feel the Sun, the Moon, and the stars. Feel the day and the night. Feel the dusk and the dawn. Feel the air and the rays of the air. Feel birds being embraced by you.

Feel eternal, infinite, and abundant. Bring this feeling into your entire body.

Take your time here.

Once you feel you have completed this journey, slowly deepen your breathing and bring your awareness back to your physical space.

Be gentle with yourself as you return to your normal breathing and open your eyes.

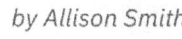

by Allison Smith

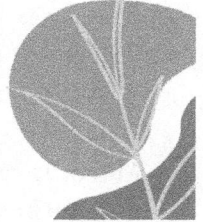

Download at *menopauseunicorn.com*

Creating Space for Connection Through Mindfulness

Mindfulness is about building the emotional strength to show up as yourself, without shame or hesitation. After I mentioned going through menopause at a Rose City Rollers event, skaters and fans alike opened up to me about their own experiences. Just sharing that I'd taken Wellbutrin was enough to make someone feel validated in their own treatment choice.

That kind of connection starts with emotional confidence. When mindfulness helps you regulate stress and quiet self-judgment, it creates the internal space to speak honestly and listen without defensiveness. It's easier to approach conversations about menopause—or any vulnerable topic—with openness and calm when you aren't carrying the weight of emotional reactivity.

Talking about menopause without shame encourages others to do the same—and those conversations are powerful. They build community, reduce isolation, and help dismantle the stigma around this phase of life. Emotional resilience gives you the freedom to be seen and understood.

Building a Sustainable Practice

Consistency is key. Meditation doesn't have to be lengthy or complicated to be effective. Try these ideas to make mindfulness part of your daily routine:

- **Morning reset:** Start your day with five minutes of mindful breathing before checking your phone.
- **Stress buffer:** When anxiety hits, pause for a one-minute body scan to release tension.
- **Evening wind-down:** Use a guided visualization before bed to ease your mind into restful sleep.

- **Anchor it:** Tie mindfulness to an existing habit—like drinking tea or brushing your teeth—to build consistency.

Mindfulness and meditation aren't quick fixes, but they are powerful tools for building emotional resilience. Over time, they help you respond with clarity rather than reacting in frustration. The result? Greater calm, more balanced emotions, and a stronger sense of control—no matter what menopause throws your way.

By creating space to breathe, reflect, and reconnect with yourself, you're building the foundation for lasting emotional wellness.

7.3 SELF-CARE STRATEGIES: PRIORITIZING YOUR WELL-BEING

Self-care isn't an indulgence—it's a survival strategy. During menopause, when your body and mind are working overtime to adjust to hormonal changes, self-care becomes essential. It's the deliberate act of refilling your emotional and physical reserves, creating a buffer against stress and helping you navigate this phase with strength and clarity. Self-care isn't about bubble baths and face masks (though those can help)—it's about recognizing what your body and mind need and responding with care and intention.

Menopause is demanding. You're facing sleep disruptions, mood swings, energy dips, and brain fog—all while managing the regular pressures of work, relationships, and daily life. Self-care gives you the tools to reset, recover, and show up as your best self. It's about reclaiming your time and energy so you can handle life's challenges from a place of strength rather than depletion.

Find What Fills You Up

The beauty of self-care lies in its diversity. For me, it often means blending movement with connection. Exercise has always been my primary act of self-care. I'm in the gym working out with friends every morning at 7 a.m. Watching the sun rise on the drive there is an added bonus—a reminder that the world is still beautiful even when life feels chaotic. The combination of movement, nature, and social connection grounds me and lifts my mood. People, exercise, and nature rule! They provide the emotional and physical foundation I need to face the day with clarity and resilience.

Take time and explore what works for you. Your version might be yoga or dancing, hiking alone, or walking with a friend. It could be a quiet moment with your coffee in the morning or listening to your favorite podcast while you garden. The key is to discover the activities that replenish your energy and make you feel grounded.

✧ **HOT TIP:** Studies have shown that regular exercise reduces cortisol levels and improves mood regulation during menopause (*Journal of Aging and Physical Activity*, 2020). Even 10 minutes of movement a day can create a noticeable shift in emotional and physical resilience.

Build Rest into Your Routine

Rest is essential, not optional. Menopause changes your sleep patterns, often making it harder to fall asleep or stay asleep. That's why it's important to create intentional rest habits that signal to your brain and body that it's time to unwind.

> "If someone's not sleeping, that's the first thing we have to tackle. It's almost impossible to feel good when you're sleep-deprived."
>
> — CHRISTINA CAMELI, CNM

For me, skincare has become a soothing nightly ritual. I layer on my lotions and potions, tackling the changes in my skin while reinforcing my commitment to care for myself. This act of winding down tells my brain it's time to shift from high gear to rest mode.

Unplugging from screens an hour before bed can also make a huge difference. Blue light from phones and TVs interferes with melatonin production, making it harder for your body to relax. Instead, opt for a book, calming music, or a gentle stretching routine. Find the rhythm that works for you.

✦ **HOT TIP:** Struggling with sleep? Try progressive muscle relaxation. Lie down, tighten each muscle group for five seconds, then release. Start at your feet and work your way up. This helps your body and mind release tension, making it easier to drift off.

Creative Nourishment Matters

Creativity is an overlooked but powerful form of self-care. When you engage in creative activities, your brain shifts from stress response to flow state, allowing you to focus and recharge. For me, it's listening to management theory audiobooks while I cook or garden—it lights me up and helps me think more clearly. For you, it could be painting, writing, knitting, or trying a new recipe.

Creativity gives your mind a break from overthinking and problem-solving. It allows you to explore, play, and create without pressure. This shift from productivity to play is essential for mental balance.

Set Boundaries Like You Mean It

One of the hardest but most impactful forms of self-care is learning to say **no**. Setting boundaries protects your energy and ensures that you're not constantly pouring from an empty cup.

As the founder and Executive Director of the Rose City Rollers, I've spent the last 20+ years being a workaholic—working 60+ hours a week, picking up the slack, and pushing through exhaustion. But menopause has made it clear: that pace is unsustainable. I've had to learn to protect my time and energy. That means turning down requests that drain me and prioritizing the things that align with my values and well-being.

Saying no isn't selfish—it's self-preservation. It allows you to protect your emotional and physical reserves so you can show up fully for the things that matter.

If you struggle with saying no, start with small boundaries: limit your availability for evening calls, say no to social obligations that feel draining, or decline extra work when your plate is already full. Boundaries create space for you to take care of yourself.

✦ **Script It:** If saying no feels uncomfortable, try this:

- "I'd love to help, but I'm at capacity right now."
- "That sounds great, but I need to protect some downtime this week."
- "I can't commit to that, but I appreciate you thinking of me."

Self-Compassion is Non-Negotiable

At the heart of self-care is self-compassion. Menopause is a vulnerable time. Your body is changing, your mood might feel unpredictable, and you may feel like you're not handling it "well enough." Self-compassion means letting go of that inner critic and meeting yourself with the same care you'd extend to a close friend.

Perfectionism has no place in self-care. Some days you'll skip the workout, miss the bedtime routine, or snap at your partner. That's normal. That's called being human. Self-compassion means accepting that missteps are part of the process and not beating yourself up for them.

Instead of thinking, *"I should have handled that better,"* try, *"I did the best I could today with the energy I had."* Reframing your inner dialogue from self-criticism to self-acceptance creates a foundation for emotional strength and resilience.

✦ **HOT TIP:** Research shows that self-compassion reduces stress, increases motivation, and improves emotional resilience (*Journal of Clinical Psychology*, 2019). Practicing positive self-talk—especially during setbacks—helps you bounce back faster and with greater confidence.

Making Self-Care a Non-Negotiable

The more you invest in your well-being, the more capable you become of handling life's curveballs. When you take time to rest, move, and nourish your body and mind, you build a foundation of resilience that allows you to thrive through menopause and beyond.

Start small. Choose one or two self-care practices that feel easy and sustainable. Gradually layer in more as you feel the benefits.

Some days, self-care might look like a long hike with a friend; other days, it might be sitting on the couch with a book and a warm blanket.

The key is consistency. Show up for yourself, day after day, in whatever way you can. Your needs matter. Your well-being matters. And taking care of yourself isn't a luxury—it's an essential part of navigating this next chapter with strength and grace. You owe it to yourself.

7.4 CREATING A MENOPAUSE JOURNAL: TRACKING YOUR JOURNEY

Journaling during menopause is a powerful tool for self-reflection, emotional processing, and symptom tracking. As menopause unfolds, it can feel like you're riding a wave of unpredictable emotions and physical shifts. A journal offers a safe, private space to process these changes and make sense of them on your terms. It's about exploring feelings, finding patterns, and empowering yourself with a deeper understanding of your body and mind.

Menopause is a time of transformation, and journaling allows you to document that process with honesty and curiosity. The simple act of slowing down and writing creates mental space. It allows you to name what's happening—to acknowledge your frustration with a sleepless night or to celebrate a day without a hot flash. This process of externalizing your thoughts fosters clarity and emotional regulation. When you journal consistently, you create a roadmap of your experience—a record that reflects not only the challenges but also the strength and growth that emerge along the way.

Why Journaling Works

Journaling engages both the logical and emotional parts of your brain, creating a bridge between thoughts and feelings. When you write down your experiences, you activate your prefrontal cortex (responsible for problem-solving and emotional regulation) while calming the amygdala (the brain's stress center). This neurological shift helps reduce anxiety and improve emotional clarity.

Research supports the benefits of expressive writing, particularly for women navigating hormonal shifts. A 2021 study in *The Journal of Psychosomatic Research* found that journaling about stressful experiences significantly reduced cortisol levels and improved mood stability. Another study published in *Menopause* in 2020 showed that symptom journaling helped women identify patterns and triggers, leading to more effective symptom management.

Journaling is also a form of mindfulness. It roots you in the present moment, while giving you the tools to process the past and prepare for the future. It transforms abstract emotions into something tangible and manageable. By naming your feelings, you create a sense of control rather than feeling overwhelmed by the chaos of hormonal change.

What to Write: Prompts to Inspire Insight

Staring at a blank page can feel intimidating, especially when you're already feeling overwhelmed. The key is to keep it simple and start where you are. Here are some easy prompts to help you begin:

Daily Reflections:

- What's one thing I'm grateful for today?
- How am I feeling physically and emotionally right now?
- What's one small win I experienced today?
- What's one thing I learned about myself this week?

Symptom Tracking:

- How did I sleep last night?
- Did I experience any hot flashes or mood swings today?
- What did I eat today, and how did it make me feel?
- Did stress feel manageable or overwhelming today?

Emotional Processing:

- What's one fear I have about menopause, and how can I reframe it?
- What's a recent moment of joy I experienced?
- What's one piece of advice I'd give my younger self about this phase of life?

Empowerment:

- What's something I'm proud of?
- How is this phase of life shaping the women I'm becoming?
- What does strength look like for me today?

Future-Focused:

- What's one thing I'm looking forward to?
- How do I want to feel next week, and what can I do to make that happen?
- What's one self-care practice I'd like to try?

✦ **HOT TIP:** Try setting a timer for 5–10 minutes and writing continuously without editing or censoring yourself. The goal isn't perfection—it's self-expression.

Track Patterns to Take Back Control

Journaling isn't just about emotional processing. It's also a practical tool for symptom tracking and pattern recognition. When you document physical changes like sleep disturbances, mood swings, and hot flashes, you start to see connections:

- Are certain foods triggering night sweats?
- Does exercise improve your mood or make you feel more fatigued?
- Are your symptoms worse during stressful weeks?

This information allows you to make informed adjustments to your lifestyle, diet, and even medication. Tracking patterns over time gives you a clearer picture of your body's needs—and helps you feel more in control of the changes happening within you.

◈ **Example:** After tracking for a month, you might notice that having caffeine after noon triggers poor sleep or that yoga reduces the intensity of your hot flashes. These insights can help you make smarter choices about how to support your body.

Make It Creative and Personal

Your journal should feel like a reflection of *you*. Some people prefer structured bullet-point lists, while others thrive on freeform writing. The format doesn't matter as long as it works for you.

- **Use Color and Texture:** Add colorful pens, stickers, or washi tape to make your journal visually appealing.
- **Include Art and Doodles:** Sketch out emotions or create mandalas as a form of stress relief.
- **Attach Photos and Mementos:** Tape in pictures from memorable events, ticket stubs, or pressed flowers from a favorite walk.
- **Create a Vision Board:** Use tools like Canva to design a board of your goals and inspirations, then attach it to the inside cover as a daily reminder of your direction.

One creative boost I found particularly empowering was using Canva to design a vision board for my 2025 goals. The process of visually mapping out my dreams felt intentional, turning abstract ideas into concrete plans. Printing this board and attaching it to the inside cover of my journal transformed it into a powerful visual anchor I return to each week for focus and inspiration.

The goal isn't to create a "perfect" journal—it's to create a personal space where you can reflect, dream, and stay grounded.

Use a Journal Designed for Menopause

If you'd rather use a structured format, there are some fantastic journals designed specifically for menopause:

- **One Line a Day** – A fan favorite! This simple journal encourages you to write just one line each day, helping you build a consistent reflection habit without feeling overwhelmed.
- **The Menopause Journal** – A guided journal with specific menopause-related prompts and symptom trackers.
- **Day One Journal** (App) – A digital option that allows you to log daily reflections and patterns, with the ability to attach photos and track data over time.
- **Five-Minute Journal** – Focuses on gratitude and positive affirmations, perfect for boosting emotional resilience.

✦ **HOT TIP:** Try keeping your journal on your nightstand and writing before bed or first thing in the morning. Creating a consistent habit helps make journaling a natural part of your routine.

Turning Journaling into a Daily Ritual

Journaling works best when it becomes a consistent habit. Even five minutes a day can make a difference. Find a time that works for you—first thing in the morning, during lunch, or right before bed—and stick with it.

Here's how to make it a habit:

- **Link it to an existing routine:** Write after brushing your teeth or while drinking your morning coffee.

- **Set a reminder:** A simple phone alert or Post-It note can keep you on track.
- **Don't overthink it:** Your entries don't need to be deep or profound. Sometimes a quick "Today was hard. Tomorrow will be better" is enough.

Your Journal, Your Journey

Your journal isn't just a record—it's a roadmap of your menopause experience. Over time, it will reflect the resilience and growth you've built along the way. It will show you how you've faced challenges, celebrated wins, and adapted with grace. When you look back months or years from now, you'll see how far you've come—and how capable you are of handling whatever comes next.

Journaling honors your real experience with honesty and care. So grab that pen and start writing. You're creating a legacy of strength and self-discovery.

7.5 THE ART OF LETTING GO: EMBRACING CHANGE AND TRANSFORMATION

Menopause is a reckoning. It's an emotional and psychological recalibration. Your body changes, your roles shift, and the familiar version of yourself may feel like it's slipping away. That loss of control—over your body, your emotions, and your identity—can feel disorienting and uncomfortable. But within this discomfort lies an incredible opportunity: the chance to redefine who you are and step into a version of yourself that's more aligned with your truth.

See this phase of your life as a time of expansion. Menopause clears away the noise and asks you to get honest about what you truly want. It strips away the societal expectations of who you're "supposed" to be and offers you the freedom to decide what comes next. But embracing that freedom requires you to release old narratives—about youth, beauty, productivity, and identity—and make room for something new.

Reframing Menopause as a Beginning, Not an End

Let's be honest—menopause often gets framed as a period of decline. The loss of fertility, the changes in appearance, the increased need for rest—all of it can feel like a slow fade-out. But that narrative is flawed. Menopause isn't a curtain call. It's the start of Act Two.

Instead of focusing on what you're losing, shift your perspective toward what you're gaining: freedom from the hormonal rollercoaster of your reproductive years, more time and space to focus on your passions, and the confidence that comes from lived experience. The person you're becoming isn't smaller or diminished. She's sharper, stronger, wiser, courageous, and more intentional.

What passions have you set aside? What dreams have you been too busy—or too scared—to pursue? Menopause creates the space to explore these questions. Maybe it's finally learning to play guitar, starting a business, or dedicating more time to travel. Or maybe it's as simple as learning to rest without guilt.

✦ **Example:** A friend of mine always dreamed of learning to surf but kept telling herself she was "too old." At 55, she finally took her first lesson—and loved it. Menopause helped her realize that age isn't a barrier; it's a reason to stop putting things off.

Discovering Who You Are Now

For me, running the Rose City Rollers has been a defining part of my life. Building the world's largest roller derby league from the ground up shaped not only my career but also my identity. But as menopause hit, I found myself asking: *Is this enough?*

The truth was, my work—while deeply fulfilling—wasn't the whole picture of who I was. Writing this book became part of my answer. It gave me a creative outlet and reminded me that I'm not just a leader and organizer. I'm also a writer, a thinker, and a creator. Menopause made me brave enough to ask: *What else?*

That's the gift of this phase—you get to redefine yourself. Your identity isn't fixed, and you're not obligated to keep doing things just because you always have. Maybe you've built a career that no longer fits. Maybe your social circle feels stale. Maybe you've been holding onto habits, relationships, or routines that don't serve you anymore. Menopause is the invitation to release those things and try something new.

Letting Go of Old Narratives

Growth requires letting go of what is no longer serving you and making space for new ideas and passions. That means releasing the outdated stories you've told yourself about who you are and what you're capable of.

- *I'm too old to start over.*
- *I should have it all figured out by now.*
- *I'm not attractive anymore.*
- *I have to keep doing what's expected of me.*

These are just stories—not facts. Menopause is the perfect time to rewrite them. The world often treats women as though they lose value as they age—but that's society's problem, not yours. There's nothing more powerful than a woman who knows her worth and owns her choices.

Start small. If you've always been the one who says yes to everything, practice saying no. If you've been clinging to a role that no longer fits, give yourself permission to step away. If you've been defining yourself by your appearance, your productivity, or your relationships—start asking who you are beyond those things.

✦ **HOT TIP:** Try a "letting go" ceremony. Write down the stories or beliefs that are no longer serving you, then burn them, rip them up, or toss them into the ocean. Symbolic gestures can make the emotional shift feel more real.

Celebrate the Wins

Menopause is hard—and you deserve to celebrate every step forward. Create rituals that mark your progress and honor your growth:

- **Host a menopause milestone party.** Gather your closest friends and celebrate the strength it takes to face this transition with grace.
- **Create a personal victory list.** Write down every small win—whether it's finding a supplement that helps you sleep better or getting through a week without a mood swing.
- **Take yourself out for a treat.** When you hit a milestone—like sticking to a meditation routine or nailing a difficult conversation—celebrate it.

These celebrations aren't frivolous—they're affirmations. They remind you that you're capable, resilient, and evolving.

What Letting Go Actually Feels Like

Letting go is a practice. Some days you'll feel light and free; other days you'll feel nostalgic for the person you used to be. That's normal.

But the more you lean into this transition with curiosity rather than resistance, the more you'll discover how expansive this phase of life can be. You are not fading. You are not shrinking. You are stepping into a version of yourself that's stronger, more confident, and more fully aligned with who you truly are.

Menopause is the beginning of a new chapter—and you get to write it exactly the way you want.

Embracing Emotional and Mental Wellness

KEY Takeaways

1. Mood swings, rage, and brain fog are real and hormone-driven.
2. Therapy, movement, and mindfulness help your emotional health.
3. You are not alone—talking about it lifts shame and creates support.

HOT TIPs

- 💎 CBT-M + movement + meds = a smarter support plan.
- 💎 Move your body daily—even 10 minutes counts.
- 💎 Talk openly about mood changes with friends and providers.

ACTION ITEMS

- ☐ Track emotional symptoms for 30 days—note patterns and triggers.
- ☐ Try guided meditation, journaling, or EMDR therapy.
- ☐ Make a list of daily habits that help you feel emotionally grounded.
- ☐ Reach out to a therapist or menopause-informed coach.

✦ Resources ✦

- App: Insight Timer
- Book: The Upgrade by Louann Brizendine
- Instagram: @drtaniaglyde
- Podcast: Therapy Chat with Laura Reagan

NEXT UP — *Chapter 8 turns the spotlight on intimacy, relationships, and reimagining connection as your body and needs evolve.*

8

REVITALIZING RELATIONSHIPS AND INTIMACY

8.1 LOVE IN THE TIME OF MENOPAUSE: NURTURING RELATIONSHIPS

Menopause changes more than just your body. It shifts the dynamics of your closest relationships. The emotional swings, physical discomfort, and mental fog can create quiet distance even in the strongest partnerships. You might feel disconnected from your partner without knowing exactly why. They might sense the change too but hesitate to bring it up, unsure how to offer support.

It's not just about intimacy—it's about feeling seen and understood. When your body feels unpredictable, even small things like planning a date night or engaging in physical affection can feel overwhelming. But rebuilding connection during menopause isn't about grand gestures—it's about consistent, meaningful moments of presence and understanding.

Build Connection Through Small Moments

Setting aside quality time together can be a surprisingly powerful way to stay connected. It doesn't have to be elaborate—a weekly date night, a morning coffee together, or an evening walk can create pockets of connection. The key is to be fully present. Put away phones, pause the mental to-do list, and focus on each other.

One thing that's worked well for my husband and me is setting dates on the calendar for small house projects. There's something grounding about working on a shared investment and building a future together—especially at a time when my body (and the world) can feel pretty out of control. Painting a room, organizing a closet, or tackling the garden can help you and your partner feel like a team. And feeling like you have control over something, no matter how small, helps balance the chaos menopause can bring.

Active listening is another underrated superpower. When your partner is speaking, don't just listen to the words—pay attention to the emotions behind them. Reflect back what you hear and try to understand their perspective without immediately jumping in to fix things. That kind of mutual effort helps bridge emotional gaps and builds deeper intimacy.

Try New Things Together

Shared activities can help rekindle a sense of adventure and discovery. My husband and I are building a new garden on our property right now with the goal of slashing our food budget, canning a ton of food, and freeze-drying even more. It's exciting to dream together about how this will pay off down the road, but I'll be honest—working together during menopause isn't always easy.

I'm bossy by nature, and menopause has made me more reactive at times. There have been moments when I've had to consciously let him do things his way, even when my instinct was to micromanage. Sometimes I've had to remind myself that hormones are making me more critical, and that letting go is better for our relationship. And honestly? It's been worth it. Watching our progress and knowing we've built something together makes the effort meaningful.

Enrolling in a cooking class, tackling a home project, or trying a new hiking trail are all ways to build new memories. These shared experiences create a sense of teamwork and remind you that you're still a unit, facing life's changes side by side.

Teamwork Is Everything

Navigating menopause as a team means developing a shared plan for symptom management and emotional support. Talk openly about what's working and where you need more help. Maybe your partner can adjust their schedule to give you time to rest or step in when you need a break. Support each other's personal growth, too. Encourage hobbies or passions, even if it means stepping outside your comfort zone to attend a partner's art show or fitness class.

Celebrate the small wins. Did you sleep through the night? That's a win. Did you both manage to stay patient during a tough moment? Another win. Acknowledging progress builds confidence and helps you both feel like you're in this together.

✧ Interactive Element: "Revitalize Together" Checklist

This checklist is a guide to nurturing your relationship during menopause, emphasizing connection and mutual support. Try to incorporate one or two items each week and adjust as needed.

- **Weekly Date Night:** Schedule a standing date night and rotate who plans the activity. Keep it simple and low-pressure, like a movie night at home or trying a new recipe.
- **Active Listening Exercise:** Set aside 10 minutes each week where one partner speaks without interruption, and the other listens fully. Then switch. Reflect back what you hear.
- **Shared Hobby Exploration:** Choose a new hobby to explore together—a cooking class, a puzzle night, or weekend gardening. Keep it light and fun.
- **House Project:** Choose a small project to work on together—painting a room, reorganizing a closet, or building a garden. Focus on collaboration, not perfection.
- **Weekly Check-In:** Have a low-stakes, honest conversation about how you're both feeling. Celebrate wins and adjust plans as needed.
- **Encourage Personal Growth:** Support each other's interests, even when they're outside your comfort zone. Show up for each other's wins.

8.2 HONEST CONVERSATIONS: TALKING ABOUT MENOPAUSE WITH PARTNERS

Talking about menopause with your partner can feel daunting, but it's also one of the most important steps toward building understanding and support. It's easy to assume that your partner will notice the changes you're going through, but unless you spell it out, they might not connect the dots.

A simple opening like, *"I've been going through some changes lately, and I'd love to share what that's been like for me,"* can be a gentle way to start the conversation. You don't need to have all the answers. Simply being honest about what you're experiencing can help your partner feel more included in the process. Share what a typical day feels like for you: the mental fog, the emotional swings, the physical discomfort, and even the surprising wins (like sleeping through the night). Transparency builds empathy, and when your partner understands the emotional and physical realities of menopause, they can better show up for you.

Education Builds Empathy

It's hard for your partner to support you if they don't understand what's happening—and that's not their fault. Menopause isn't exactly well-covered in health class. Offering resources can help bridge that knowledge gap. You could share:

- An article or book about the science of menopause
- A podcast episode or YouTube video that explains the symptoms in a relatable way
- A social media post from a menopause doctor that reflects your experience

Encourage your partner to ask questions, even the ones that feel awkward or uninformed. A question like *"Is it normal to have brain fog?"* or *"Why does menopause affect sleep?"* isn't silly. It's a chance to clear up misconceptions and strengthen your connection. If they feel comfortable asking questions, you've created a safe space where learning and growth are possible.

Navigating Sensitive Topics

Changes in libido, mood swings, and emotional distance can be harder to discuss. The key is timing and tone. Don't try to have a heavy conversation when one of you is exhausted, distracted, or emotionally overwhelmed. Choose a calm moment when you're both relaxed. Ask your partner if they have the bandwidth for the conversation.

Start with *"I've noticed..."* or *"I've been feeling...",* rather than *"You never..."* or *"Why don't you..."* This keeps the conversation from feeling like an attack. Focus on how you feel rather than what they might be doing wrong. For example:

- *"I've been feeling disconnected lately, and I think part of it is how menopause is affecting my energy."*
- *"Sometimes I feel emotionally distant, and I don't want you to think it's about you."*
- *"I've been going through some changes, and I'm still figuring out how to talk about them."*
- *"This might come out a little messy, but I want to be honest about what I'm feeling."*

If the conversation starts to feel tense, take a break. A simple, *"Let's come back to this tomorrow when we're both feeling more clearheaded,"* can help reset the tone. Remember, you don't need to solve everything in one sitting.

Teamwork and Gratitude Matter

Mutual support and empathy are the bedrock of a strong relationship during menopause. It's easy to focus on what's hard, but focusing on what's working can shift the dynamic. Expressing gratitude for small things—like when your partner brings you a glass of water during a hot flash or patiently listens when you vent—reinforces the idea that you're in this together.

One thing my husband and I have found helpful is thanking each other, even for the small stuff. It sounds cheesy, but just saying *"Thanks for being patient with me today"* or *"I appreciate you checking in with me"* goes a long way in feeling supported.

Support isn't always about grand gestures. Sometimes it's just sitting next to each other in silence or holding hands during a rough moment. Let your partner know that just being there matters.

✦ Interactive Element: Conversation Starters

These prompts can help guide an open, low-stakes conversation about menopause. Try starting with one or two and see where it leads:

- *"Can I tell you a little about what menopause has been like for me?"*
- *"I've been feeling off lately. Can we talk about how this is affecting us?"*
- *"Do you want to know more about the symptoms I've been experiencing?"*
- *"How have you been feeling about the changes we've been going through?"*
- *"What's one way I can help you feel more connected right now?"*

✦ **HOT TIPs:**

- **Timing matters:** Don't start heavy conversations when one of you is tired, hungry, or distracted.
- **Avoid blame:** Focus on "I" statements to avoid defensiveness.
- **Be specific:** Instead of *"You don't care,"* say, *"I feel disconnected when we don't spend time together."*
- **Take breaks if needed:** If the conversation gets heated, step away and revisit it later.

8.3 SEXUAL HEALTH: ADDRESSING CHANGES AND ENHANCING PLEASURE

Sexual health during menopause isn't just about desire—it's about connection.

Menopause changes how you experience intimacy, both physically and emotionally. Decreased estrogen levels can lead to vaginal dryness, reduced sensitivity, and a dip in desire. But even more than the physical changes, the emotional shifts—feeling disconnected from your body, your partner, or yourself—can make intimacy feel more like a chore than a source of connection.

But here's the truth: intimacy isn't just about sex—it's about feeling valued, connected, and comfortable in your skin. Rediscovering pleasure starts with understanding your body's new responses and communicating openly with your partner.

Rebuilding Intimacy Through Connection

Desire doesn't always show up on cue, especially during menopause. Emotional connection often precedes physical desire, so if you're feeling disconnected from your partner, rebuilding that emotional bridge is the first step.

- **Start small.** Physical touch doesn't have to lead to sex. Holding hands, cuddling on the couch, or giving a back massage creates closeness without pressure.
- **Practice vulnerability.** Sharing how you're feeling—both physically and emotionally—creates intimacy. Saying *"I've been feeling disconnected lately; I'd love to feel closer to you"* opens the door to deeper connection.
- **Redefine intimacy.** Sometimes, sexual connection is about exploring what feels good now, which doesn't always lead to intercourse. Mutual massage, oral sex, or simply taking more time to explore each other's bodies can shift the focus from performance to pleasure.

Create a New Sexual Blueprint

Menopause is the perfect time to explore what feels good *now*—because it might be different than what felt good in your 30s.

- Try new positions or different types of touch.
- Incorporate vibrators or toys if it enhances sensation.
- Focus on pleasure, not orgasm—sometimes the goal is relaxation and closeness.

Sensory experiences—like warm oils, scented candles, and soft textures—can help you reconnect with your body and enhance physical connection.

Managing Expectations and Frustration

Not every attempt at intimacy will be perfect—and that's okay. Some nights you'll feel into it; other nights, you won't. That doesn't mean you're losing your connection.

Be honest with your partner about what feels good and what doesn't. If you need to stop or shift gears, say so. Sexual connection is about mutual enjoyment. There's no script you need to follow.

Here are some ideas to get things flowing.

- **Create a pleasure menu:** List activities that feel good, from cuddling to oral sex, and explore them together without pressure.
- **Take the pressure off orgasm:** Focus on sensation and pleasure rather than a specific outcome.
- **Use humor:** Laughter can dissolve tension and bring you closer together.

When More Support is Needed

If you're feeling disconnected or frustrated, a sex therapist can help guide you through these changes. They can offer techniques for building desire and improving communication. Books like *Come as You Are* by Emily Nagoski and *Mating in Captivity* by Esther Perel can also help you rethink sexual intimacy and rediscover pleasure.

8.4 RECONNECTING WITH YOURSELF: SELF-EXPLORATION AND CONFIDENCE

For years, you've likely poured energy into everyone else—partners, kids, work, family, and friends. But menopause changes the game. It's about realizing that you don't have to keep showing up for everyone else at the expense of yourself.

This is your moment to reclaim your time, your body, and your sense of self. And here's the best part: you've earned the right to stop giving so many fucks. This isn't about being selfish—it's about survival. The people who love you will adjust. The ones who don't? That's not your problem.

Menopause strips away the noise—the need to please, the pressure to meet expectations. What's left is the opportunity to rebuild a life that actually works for you.

Rediscover What Feels Good

Menopause gives you the rare chance to ask yourself: *What do I actually want?*

After years of being a caregiver, a professional, a partner, or a parent, you finally have the space to rediscover yourself outside of those roles. Allow yourself to ask the questions and be open to any kind of answer:

- What lights me up now?
- What relationships feel nourishing—and which ones drain me?
- What's one thing I'm ready to stop doing?

Journaling is a powerful way to tap into this self-exploration. You don't need to sit down and write an emotional manifesto—just start with simple prompts:

- What would a perfect day look like?
- If no one else's needs mattered, how would I spend my time?
- What's one thing I've always wanted to try but never did?

And then—start trying things. But skip the boring, predictable stuff. Find what truly makes you feel alive.

- Take an adult trampoline class and laugh until your sides hurt.
- Try pole dancing—it's empowering, playful, and a killer workout.
- Learn how to throw axes—because sometimes you just need to smash things.
- Start a monthly dinner club where everyone has to cook something new.
- Go to a punk show and stand near the front. Feel the music vibrate through you.
- Volunteer with your local roller derby league—because it's badass, supportive, and wildly fun.

The goal is about exploration. You don't need to become an expert. Reconnect with your inner child, with your imagination, and let yourself play.

Rebuilding Confidence—Inside and Out

Menopause changes your body, and that shift can mess with your self-image. But here's the truth: confidence is about how you feel in your skin, not how you look.

I recently found myself in a major clothing rut after losing 60 pounds. My clothes felt frumpy, and honestly, I had no idea what to wear as the world was coming out of COVID and I was heading into perimenopause. I remembered that I've always loved a low-cut shirt with a bit of cleavage, so I pulled out some of my old favorites. But my jeans were bagging in a not-so-cute way, so I did some research and found modern cuts that work with my size 14/16 hourglass figure.

Game. Changer.

Suddenly, I felt like *me* again. And here's the thing: confidence radiates. When you feel good in your clothes, it changes the way you move through the world.

And social media? It's full of Gen Xers rediscovering their style and leaning into this new phase with zero shame. Seeing other women my age owning their looks reminded me that this phase is about showing up as the boldest version of yourself.

Find what makes you feel good—whether that's investing in new jeans that fit right or embracing bold lipstick. It's not vanity—it's self-respect.

Reclaim Your Time and Energy

One of the greatest gifts of menopause is realizing that you can say no without apology.

If you don't want to go to the family dinner, *don't go.*

If you're exhausted and someone asks you for a favor, *say no.*

If someone asks why you're stepping back, *you don't owe them an explanation.*

When you stop overexplaining and justifying, you reclaim so much energy. You're no longer managing other people's feelings or trying to keep everyone happy. And the people who truly care about you will adjust. The ones who don't? Adios!

Let Go of the Bullshit

This is the time to release the pressure to be everything to everyone. It's okay to outgrow friendships, shift your priorities, and leave behind the version of yourself that no longer fits.

You don't have to stay the same just to make other people comfortable.

- If you're not into small talk anymore, skip the social gathering.
- If your friends are pressuring you to keep up the same routine—set a boundary.
- If someone is making you feel guilty for choosing yourself—walk away.

You've earned the right to take up space. To speak your mind. To try something new—and maybe even suck at it without caring. To live according to your values without asking for permission.

Menopause strips away the need to please—and what's left is the real you. Stronger, bolder, and more in tune with what you actually want.

Own it, you badass.

8.5 NAVIGATING FAMILY DYNAMICS: SHARING YOUR EXPERIENCE

You walk through the door after a long day, and chaos greets you like an old friend. Normally, you'd dive right in—solving problems, breaking up arguments, answering the inevitable, *"What's for dinner?"* But today? You're running on empty. The noise, the questions, the expectations—it's all just... *too much.*

Menopause has a way of shaking up not just your relationship with yourself, but also your interactions with the people closest to you. Mood swings can turn a simple conversation into a powder keg. Brain fog might leave you forgetting why you walked into a room—or why you agreed to host Thanksgiving. Your patience wears thin, and your energy for household roles dwindles. And sometimes, the people around you don't get it—or worse, they take it personally.

It's not just you adjusting to menopause—it's your whole family. And that requires some recalibration.

Shifting Family Roles

If you've always been the emotional anchor and the household manager, menopause forces a hard reset. You simply can't run the show 24/7 anymore. And honestly? You shouldn't have to.

This is the time to redistribute emotional and physical labor within the family. If you've been carrying the mental load for years—meal planning, scheduling, remembering dentist appointments—it's time to hand some of that off.

- If your kids are old enough to drive, they're old enough to run errands.
- If your partner's been "helping" by asking what needs to be done—hand them a list.

- If your parents are relying on you for emotional support when you're barely holding it together—set a boundary.

Menopause is a shared experience, not a journey to navigate alone.

- If your kids are old enough, ask them to help with more household responsibilities.
- Encourage family members to read about menopause so they understand the physical and emotional shifts you're going through.
- Schedule a low-stakes family meeting to talk about what's working and what's not. It's not about blaming anyone—it's about adjusting together.

You don't have to be the one holding it all together anymore. Let your family meet you halfway.

And when someone asks why you're stepping back? You don't need to over-explain.

"I'm focusing on my health right now."

That's it. That's the whole sentence.

Let them figure it out. You're not responsible for managing everyone else's emotions anymore.

Talking to Your Kids

Your kids—whether they're toddlers, teenagers, or adults—might not notice the changes you're going through, but they'll *feel* them. Mood swings, fatigue, and emotional overwhelm are hard to hide from the people you live with.

If your kids are younger, keep it simple:

- *"Mom's body is going through some changes, so I might be more tired than usual. It's nothing to worry about."*
- *"If I'm a little grumpy, it's not your fault. I just need some quiet time."*

If your kids are older, give them more context:

- *"I'm going through menopause, which is basically puberty in reverse. It's normal, but it's not always fun."*
- *"Sometimes I need more space or quiet, but it doesn't mean I'm mad at you."*
- *"If I snap at you, it's probably my hormones. Let's just call a timeout and reset."*

Teenagers, in particular, are in their own hormonal chaos, so framing menopause as a natural phase (like puberty) helps normalize it without overexplaining.

And if they see you modeling self-care—setting boundaries, prioritizing rest—they'll learn that taking care of yourself is normal and healthy.

Normalize Menopause for Future Generations

One of the most valuable things you can do for your family—and for future generations—is to normalize talking about menopause.

When your daughters grow up knowing that half the population experiences menopause, they won't feel blindsided when it's their turn. And your sons will grow into compassionate men who understand that this is a natural, challenging phase—not something to mock, minimize, or ignore.

Talking openly about menopause helps future adults show up with more understanding and care for their partners, friends, and colleagues. So really, sharing your menopause journey isn't just helping you—it's shaping a more compassionate future.

Go you.

Reflecting on My Own Family Experience

I remember how menopause was a mystery when my mom went through it. The lack of understanding often led to moments of chaos, where the unpredictability of her moods caught us off guard. She would sometimes tell us to run for cover on her rough days, and while we laugh about it now, it's a reminder of how far we've come.

Today, we have a wealth of resources and support networks to draw from, making menopause a more manageable and less isolating experience. Open communication, healthy boundaries, and a supportive family environment make all the difference.

Menopause doesn't have to be a period of upheaval. It can be an opportunity to deepen family relationships—turning those "run for cover" moments into opportunities for connection and understanding.

8.6 EMPTY NEST AND BEYOND: REDEFINING YOUR ROLE

As your children step out into the world, the echo of their absence can fill your home with a strange and contradictory mix of emotions. Relief and loneliness. Freedom and uncertainty. The quietness that once seemed elusive now stretches out, offering both space and silence.

For years, your life may have revolved around school schedules, sports practices, meal planning, and last-minute emergencies. Now, without those daily demands, it's easy to feel unmoored—like you've lost part of your identity. But with this emptiness comes an opportunity: a blank canvas inviting you to rediscover what life looks like when you're not managing someone else's schedule.

This is your moment to redefine your purpose—not just as a parent, but as a person.

Embracing the Quiet

The sudden stillness after your kids leave home can feel overwhelming. The background noise of life—the chatter, the footsteps, the sound of keys in the door—disappears almost overnight.

It's tempting to fill that quiet with busywork—projects, social events, and endless to-do lists—but leaning into the quiet can be surprisingly healing. Instead of resisting it, try sitting with it. Let the silence settle in. You don't need to rush to fill the space.

- Sit on the porch with a glass of wine and just breathe.
- Read a book without interruption.
- Take a solo walk and let your mind wander.

Silence is space, not emptiness. And in that space, you get to figure out what feels good now.

And hey—if the silence isn't working for you that day? Crank up the Ramones (or Taylor Swift) and rock out while cleaning the kitchen or doing something that makes you happy. Quiet's great—but sometimes you just need to scream, *"I Wanna Be Sedated."*

Redefining Your Purpose

After years of focusing on your kids' needs, shifting that focus to yourself can feel strange—but also liberating.

This is the time to pursue things that got put on the back burner:

- Sign up for that writing workshop you've been eyeing for years.
- Finally learn to play guitar or take up pottery.
- Go back to school or explore a career shift.
- Travel solo—or take that bucket list trip with a friend.

Focus on returning to the parts of yourself that got buried under the weight of daily life.

When my mom became an empty nester, she fell back in love with painting. And it turns out, she's *unbelievably* talented. I've found myself wondering if she could've been a famous artist instead of a data analyst and professional food taste tester (yes, that was her actual job). She's not interested in chasing fame, but the joy of creating again has been enough to make this phase feel like a new beginning for her.

And if purpose for you means connection, there are plenty of ways to find it:

- Volunteering for a cause you care about (like your local roller derby league!).
- Mentoring someone younger in your field.
- Joining a book club or a community group.

Purpose doesn't have to be grand—it's about finding what makes you feel engaged and energized.

Rebuilding Adult Relationships

Parent-child relationships naturally shift as your kids step into adulthood. The challenge is figuring out how to support them without falling back into the role of caretaker.

- Respect their independence. They don't need you to manage their lives anymore.
- Offer advice when it's welcomed, not when it's assumed.
- Make space for them to share what's going on in their lives without judgment or problem-solving.
- Keep the lines of communication open—regular calls, texts, or visits—but let them take the lead sometimes.

This phase is about transitioning from being their manager to being their ally. Let them figure things out, make mistakes, and find their footing. You've given them the tools—they'll use them when they're ready.

Explore New Relationships

Without the structure of family obligations, you might notice shifts in your social life. Friendships that once revolved around your kids' activities may fade—and that's okay. This is a chance to build relationships based on shared interests and genuine connection.

- Join a hiking or walking group.
- Take a cooking class or a wine-tasting course.
- Find local events that align with your interests—art shows, trivia nights, live music.
- If you're single, you might even consider dating again—if that sounds fun.

This is about reconnecting with people who bring energy and ease into your life. Look for people who make you laugh and feel seen—and give yourself permission to walk away from those who don't.

Celebrate the Wins

Recognize and celebrate the small victories along the way:

- Learning how to use power tools? That's a win.
- Taking yourself out to dinner—and actually enjoying it? Win.
- Getting through a weekend without overthinking or overcommitting? Huge win.

Treat yourself when you hit a milestone. Buy the shoes. Open the champagne. Book the massage. You've spent years showing up for other people. Now it's time to celebrate yourself.

It's Not an Ending—It's a Reset

This phase is expansion, not loss. You've spent years defining yourself in relation to others: partner, parent, friend, colleague. Now it's about defining yourself on your own terms.

You don't have to rush to figure it all out. Just start small. Try things. Let yourself be curious. The best part? There's no deadline, no scorecard—just the quiet thrill of figuring out who you are now.

This is the start of the most interesting chapter yet. Let's go.

Revitalizing Relationships and Intimacy

8

KEY Takeaways

1. Menopause impacts emotional and physical intimacy in real ways.
2. Communication and curiosity create deeper connection.
3. Pleasure evolves — and can become even more powerful.

HOT TIPs

◈ Drop the goals and focus on shared experience.

◈ Schedule connection time without pressure.

◈ Address vaginal dryness or pain— it's treatable and common.

ACTION ITEMS

☐ Start a low-pressure conversation about emotional or physical needs.

☐ Plan one playful or sensory-focused connection experience.

☐ Try a new type of touch, massage, or shared laughter practice.

☐ Reflect on what intimacy means to you now versus ten years ago.

✦ **Resources** ✦

- Web: The Gottman Institute blog
- Book: Come As You Are by Emily Nagoski
- Instagram: @mysexbio
- Podcast: Where Should We Begin? with Esther Perel

NEXT UP

Chapter 9 is your personal power-up— harnessing this transition to fuel growth, purpose, and joy.

9

THRIVING THROUGH PERSONAL GROWTH AND TRANSFORMATION

You've made it. After navigating the twists and turns of menopause, you've arrived at a place where reinvention isn't just possible—it's inevitable. This chapter is about owning that transformation. You've done the hard work of understanding your body, recalibrating your health, and reclaiming your sense of self. Now it's time to channel that strength into thriving.

In the pages ahead, we'll explore what it means to grow into this next phase of life with purpose and audacity. You'll discover the joy of stepping into new passions, setting meaningful goals, and building resilience from the inside out. We'll celebrate the milestones you've already reached—and the ones still ahead. Most importantly, we'll talk about how to share your hard-won wisdom with the next generation, ensuring that this collective knowledge becomes a gift that keeps giving.

"We don't need more fear-mongering about menopause. This transition has so much potential—to reconnect with our bodies, learn what makes us feel good, and embrace a new, powerful phase of life."

— CHRISTINA CAMELI, CNM

9.1 EMBRACING NEW PASSIONS: FINDING JOY IN REINVENTION

Menopause is an open invitation to grow, evolve, and explore. Imagine standing at the edge of a blank canvas, not with uncertainty, but with the thrill of possibility. This is the moment to paint a new picture of who you are and who you want to become. You now have the freedom to expand into the person you were always meant to be.

And let's be real—this isn't about picking up knitting or joining a walking club (unless that lights you up). This is about saying yes to the things that scare you a little. Skydiving? Do it. Learning to surf even though you're scared of the ocean? Why not. Taking an improv class even though you might bomb the first time? That's the point. Growth isn't about comfort—it's about feeling the spark of possibility and leaning into it.

For me, writing this book has been that leap into the unknown. After 20 years of running Rose City Rollers—building a community that empowers women, girls, and nonbinary folks to find their strength on and off skates—I could have played it safe. But menopause shifted something in me. It gave me this "why the hell not" feeling. I had to learn how to self-publish, how to structure a compelling story, how to believe that I have something worth saying. The fear of failure has been both exhilarating and motivating, and honestly, I know I wouldn't have taken this on if menopause hadn't pushed me to see myself differently.

Reinvention is about letting go of the idea that you need to stay in the same lane forever. It's about trusting that you've already got the tools to tackle something unfamiliar. Learning a new skill, traveling solo, starting a business, training for a marathon —these aren't just bucket list items. They're ways to stretch your limits and see what you're capable of.

And yes, the fear will come. That little voice will tell you you're too old, too late, too out of your league. But menopause has already taught you how to push through discomfort. You've faced brain fog, weight gain, and mood swings—and you're still standing. So take the leap. Bet on yourself. That's how you build the next great chapter of your life.

You got this.

9.2 SETTING NEW GOALS: CRAFTING YOUR MENOPAUSE VISION

Menopause is the ultimate permission slip to stop chasing goals that don't serve you and start setting ones that light you up. This isn't about "having it all." It's about defining what *your* version of thriving looks like—and then going after it with purpose, tenacity, and clarity.

Focus on creating a roadmap that reflects your values and fuels your growth. And to keep you on track, we're going to tap into the SMART framework:

- **Specific** – Get clear. "Get in shape" is vague; "Deadlift 190 pounds by June" is specific.

- **Measurable** – Track your progress. If you want to save money, define how much and by when.
- **Achievable** – Stretch yourself, but don't set yourself up to fail. "Write a book" is ambitious; "Write 1,000 words a week" is achievable.
- **Relevant** – Make sure your goals align with your values and bigger life vision. If it's not meaningful to *you*, it won't stick.
- **Time-bound** – Give yourself a deadline. "Someday" is not a date.

Bringing Your Goals to Life

This is where the vision board comes in. I created one for 2025 that reflects my big goals—financial freedom, creative success, adventure, and connection. I've got images of kayaking (because I want four big adventures this year), a lush garden (because I'm committing to getting my hands dirty), and even a cheeky little note about weekly sex (because why not?). That vision board lives where I can see it every day. It's a reminder of the life I'm building—not just dreaming about.

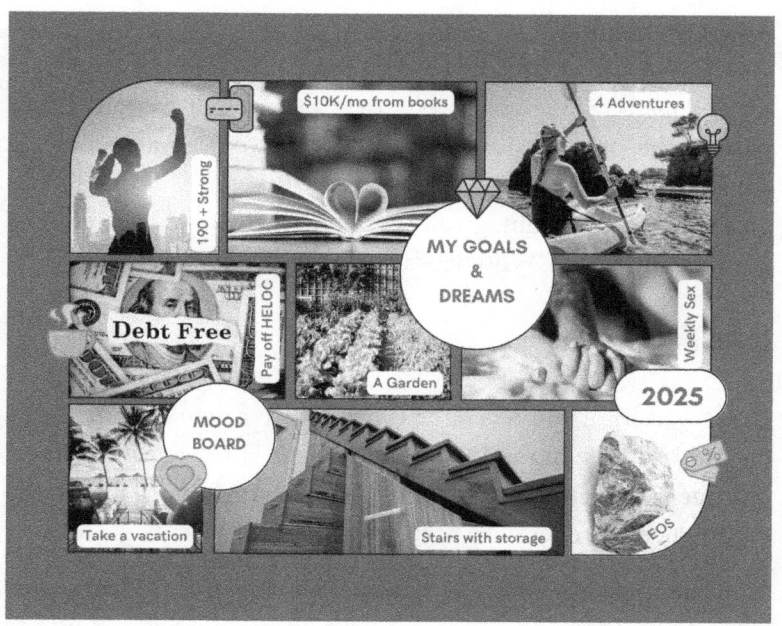

But a vision board alone won't cut it. You have to break it down into actionable steps. My goal of making $10K a month from book sales? That means setting weekly writing targets, researching marketing strategies, and tracking my progress. The kayak trip? That means looking at destinations and booking it. Big goals become real when you give them structure and momentum.

✦ HOT TIP: Make It Measurable and Visible

Take a photo of your vision board and set it as your phone background. Break each big goal down into weekly or monthly targets and write them down where you'll see them every day—on a whiteboard, in a journal, or on a sticky note next to your computer. Progress happens when you make it impossible to ignore.

Adapt and Evolve

Life happens. Some goals will stick; others will morph. That's part of the process. Flexibility is key. If you hit a roadblock, adjust—not because you failed, but because you're evolving. If a goal stops feeling right, give yourself permission to let it go. The goal is momentum. Who needs perfection?

Celebrate the Wins

Don't wait until you reach the finish line to celebrate. Finished a chapter? Treat yourself to a great meal. Hit a savings target? Splurge on a small indulgence. Those small wins build the confidence and energy to keep going.

Your menopause vision is a map to a life that reflects your strength, wisdom, and badassery. There are no right or wrong goals. Set *real* ones.. The ones that make you feel alive.

9.3 BUILDING RESILIENCE: STRENGTHENING YOUR INNER BADASS

Resilience is your armor against the unpredictability of menopause—a force that helps you navigate life's hurdles with unyielding strength. While you can't avoid being affected by these challenges, you *can* find the grit to push through them.

Resilience is the difference between getting knocked down and staying down—or getting back up and coming back stronger. During menopause, this quality becomes essential. Your body is changing, your emotions are shifting, and some days it feels like you've lost control. But resilience gives you the ability to adapt and rise above it all. It's about knowing you can handle whatever life throws your way.

Building Resilience Through Action

Developing resilience is something you cultivate through deliberate action. And here's the truth: building resilience is hard. It requires commitment and discomfort, but the payoff is undeniable strength.

Start with gratitude. Yeah, it sounds cliché, but it works. Focusing on what's going right recalibrates your mindset, helping you see solutions instead of just problems. Every day, I write down one thing I'm grateful for or send a thank-you note. (As the Executive Director of a nonprofit, there's no shortage of people to thank.) Some days, it's something big—a major win at work. Other days, it's smaller—a perfect gluten-free zucchini bread or a hilarious meme from a friend. Gratitude shifts your focus from what's hard to what's working. That shift is powerful.

Move your body. Physical resilience builds mental resilience—it's that simple. About 10 months ago, I committed to working out 5–6 days a week at 7 a.m., and I'm stronger than I've ever been. But it's not because it's been easy. My Achilles has been acting up, so I've had to modify workouts and push through setbacks.

That's resilience. It's about showing up, period. Whether you're lifting weights, pole dancing, doing Pilates, or playing roller derby (wink), movement builds strength—in your body *and* your mind.

✦ **HOT TIP:** Don't aim for consistency. Aim for adaptability. Injured? Modify. Tired? Go lighter. Don't skip—adjust. Building resilience is about learning to pivot without quitting.

Reflection = Strength

Learn from the process. Take time to reflect on what's working and what's not. When have you faced setbacks and come out stronger? What did you learn from it? For me, that's been the key to figuring out how to balance intense workouts with recovery. I don't skip—I modify. That approach has worked in business, too. Running Rose City Rollers hasn't been a smooth ride. But when things have gone sideways, I've always come back to the same process: assess, adapt, and keep moving. That's resilience.

Forget Me—Let's Talk About You

Here's the thing: you don't need an inspirational story about someone else. You already *are* the story. Every time you've gotten through a rough day, navigated a difficult relationship, or stood up for yourself when it would have been easier to stay quiet—that's resilience. Every time you've gone to a workout when you wanted to stay in bed, every time you've asked for help, every time you've pushed past discomfort—that's resilience. You already have it. Now it's about leveling up.

Resilience = Power

Grow stronger because of setbacks. Become the kind of person who knows that you can't control everything, but you can control how you respond. Menopause is going to throw some curveballs. But you're already strong enough to handle it. The key is trusting that strength, flexing it, and knowing that every time you rise, you become more unstoppable.

9.4 CELEBRATING YOUR JOURNEY: MILESTONES AND ACHIEVEMENTS

Pause for a moment. Take a breath. Look back at the winding path that brought you here. It's easy to overlook how far you've come—the setbacks you've pushed through, the growth you've fought for, the strength you've built. But recognizing personal milestones isn't just feel-good fluff—it's fuel. When you take stock of your progress, you remind yourself that you're capable of doing hard things. You see proof of your resilience. And that's what drives you forward.

Track It to Believe It

A few years ago, after one of our annual all-league meetings at Rose City Rollers—our big "Rocktober" gathering—I started hearing some well-meaning but slightly grouchy feedback: *Nothing ever comes from these meetings.* Fair enough. So we started a spreadsheet to track changes and goals that came out of Rocktober.

And guess what? The impact was massive. Seeing progress written down made it real. It turned vague hopes into measurable wins. Suddenly, we could look back and say, *Look at what we made happen.*

You can do the same with your personal goals. Keep a list, a journal, or (if you're more tech-savvy) try one of these tracking tools:

- **Notion** – Build a life dashboard with long-term and short-term goals.
- **Todoist** – Create recurring tasks and track daily progress.

- **Streaks** – Great for building consistent habits (like working out or journaling).
- **Trello** – Visualize goals on boards and move them from "To Do" to "Done."
- **Coach.me** – Set goals and track them with personal coaching support.

✦ **HOT TIP:** Take a screenshot of your goal tracker and make it your phone background. The more you see it, the more likely you are to stick with it.

Make It a Celebration

Celebrations don't have to be grand to be meaningful. Finishing a project? Go out for a cocktail (or mocktail). Hit a new personal best at the gym? Buy yourself some new workout gear. Finally finish that big work presentation? Take the day off and binge your favorite show. Small wins deserve small rewards. Big wins deserve *big* rewards. Don't be shy about celebrating your own badassery.

A personal celebration could be as simple as a solo afternoon with a good book or a long hike. Or maybe you want to gather your friends and family for a night out where you let people toast you for how hard you've worked. Whatever feels authentic—do that. The point isn't the size of the celebration; it's the acknowledgment that you *earned it*.

Share It

If you feel comfortable, share your milestones publicly. Not in a "look at me" way, but in a "look what's possible" way. Post about the goal you crushed or the challenge you pushed through. Express gratitude for the people who supported you. This isn't about curating a highlight reel. It's about owning your story and giving others permission to own theirs too.

I've shared gratitude and wins online, and I've been blown away by the response. It creates a ripple effect. Other people feel seen and inspired, and suddenly they're sharing their wins too. There's power in collective encouragement. Let's normalize cheering for ourselves—and for each other.

Your Journey = Proof of Your Strength

Every milestone you've reached, every setback you've survived, every time you've shown up for yourself—it all matters. Resilience isn't about the destination; it's about who you become on the way there. So celebrate it all. Toast your wins. Laugh off the failures. Share the lessons. Keep setting bigger, bolder goals. You've already proven you can handle the hard part. Now it's time to enjoy the ride.

9.5 THE MENOPAUSE UNICORN: THRIVING AGAINST ALL ODDS

In the midst of menopause, finding strength in our individuality can be one of the most empowering experiences. Each woman's path through menopause is unique—there's no single "right" way to navigate it. Whether you view it as a time of challenge or opportunity, embracing your own experience is key to thriving.

Reflect on your personal strengths—those qualities that have carried you through life's ups and downs. They are your allies now, more than ever. Maybe it's your resilience, your creativity, or your unwavering determination. These traits are what make you uniquely equipped to handle whatever menopause throws your way.

Mindset Matters

Maintaining a positive mindset can transform how you experience menopause. It's not always easy—brain fog and mood swings have a way of messing with your confidence—but practicing positive self-talk helps shift your perspective. Surround yourself with supportive, uplifting influences—friends, family, or even online communities that understand what you're going through. These connections can bolster your spirit and provide a network of encouragement and strength.

The power of optimism and resilience in overcoming challenges is profound. By focusing on what you can control and choosing to view your experience through a lens of possibility, you open yourself to the potential for growth and transformation. It's not about "thinking your way out" of menopause—it's about meeting the experience with strength and grace.

Proof That It's Possible

Take **Michelle Obama**. She's spoken openly about experiencing hot flashes while traveling on Air Force One and how menopause disrupted her sense of balance. But instead of letting it slow her down, she leaned into it. She focused on her health and well-being, started adjusting her workouts, and made space for self-care. She used the experience to recalibrate and came out stronger, more centered, and more self-assured. Michelle has framed menopause as a time for reclaiming personal power and redefining balance—a chance to focus on what truly matters.

Then there's **Jane Fonda**. Jane has said that post-menopause was when she found her true confidence and sense of purpose. After decades in the public eye, she finally felt free from the pressure to be "perfect." Menopause became a gateway to liberation—a time when she leaned into activism, started taking on more personal projects, and fully embraced her identity without compromise. Jane has said that physical strength and regular exercise were key to helping her navigate menopause—not just physically, but mentally and emotionally.

These are powerful testimonies of thriving. Michelle and Jane didn't *survive* menopause—they transformed through it. They treated it not as a period of decline, but as a launching pad for reinvention. Their stories remind us that menopause isn't about losing anything. It's about gaining clarity, freedom, and strength.

Your Story Matters

Sharing your story can be a powerful tool for both healing and empowerment. By opening up about your experience, you have the opportunity to inspire others and create a sense of community and belonging. Consider sharing your journey on platforms like TikTok, Instagram, or even a podcast. A short, honest post about what's worked for you (or what hasn't) can resonate with others who may feel alone or misunderstood.

Be real about your struggles and victories, about your setbacks and breakthroughs. Your story matters because it's honest—and honesty is powerful. Every time a woman talks about her experience, it chips away at the stigma and silence around menopause. It reminds others that they're not alone—and that thriving through menopause isn't just possible, it's inevitable.

You Are the Menopause Unicorn

The journey through menopause is about being real, not perfect. It's about honoring your body's changes, tapping into your inner strength, and deciding that this next chapter will be the most empowered one yet. Michelle, Jane, and countless other women have shown that menopause can be a time of reinvention and discovery. Now it's your turn. Own your experience. Share your story. And let this be the beginning of the most powerful phase of your life.

9.6 EMPOWERING THE NEXT GENERATION: SHARING YOUR WISDOM

Imagine sitting down with a younger woman—maybe a daughter, a niece, or a friend—and telling her the truth about menopause. Not the sanitized, polite version. The real stuff: the hot flashes, the brain fog, the weight gain, the hormonal chaos—but also the strength, the clarity, the freedom that comes with it. Imagine the relief on her face when she realizes she's not crazy, not broken, and not alone.

And here's the kicker: even when you've got your hormones pretty dialed in, menopause can still blindside you. I've had days where I've had to physically talk myself down from ramming my cart into people at Costco. That menopause rage? It's real. And it doesn't mean you're failing or regressing. It just means menopause is unpredictable. Some days you feel balanced and centered; other days you're two seconds from a meltdown in the frozen foods aisle. That's part of it. And that's why sharing the truth matters.

Mentorship Can Be Casual (or Not)

Mentorship doesn't have to look like a formal sit-down session over tea. It can be a casual conversation over drinks or a direct message exchange on social media. It could be a quick voice note to a younger friend saying, "Hey, I see you're struggling. This worked for me." Passing on wisdom is about showing up with honesty and vulnerability.

And it goes both ways. The younger generation has a lot to teach us too. They've grown up with language around mental health and gender identity that many of us didn't have. They know how to build online communities and normalize difficult conversations. Bridging that generational gap strengthens everyone.

Documenting Your Story = Creating a Legacy

One of the most powerful gifts you can give the next generation is your story. Not some polished, Insta-perfect version of it—the real version. The struggles, the breakthroughs, the awkward and uncomfortable parts.

Forget the "letter to your younger self." This is about creating a record that future generations can actually *use*. Start a TikTok series, create a podcast episode, or post an Instagram reel about the three things you wish you'd known before menopause hit. Hell, put it in a group chat. The medium doesn't matter. What matters is that you're capturing the truth and putting it out into the world.

✦ **HOT TIP:** Want to start small? Try recording a short voice memo about one thing that surprised you about menopause. Save it. That's your starting point for documenting your legacy.

Amplify Other Voices

You don't have to be the loudest person in the room to create a ripple effect. Sometimes the most powerful thing you can do is amplify someone else's voice. Share a post from a menopause advocate. Recommend a book or podcast that helped you. Comment on someone's experience and let them know they're not alone.

That's how communities form—through shared experiences and mutual support. Look at what's happening around reproductive health and abortion rights—grassroots conversations are driving massive cultural shifts. The same thing can happen with menopause. We just have to start talking.

Teach Them to Expect More

Part of empowering the next generation is teaching them to expect more from their healthcare, their workplaces, and their communities. Menopause support is a necessity, not a luxury. Encourage younger women to ask better questions, demand better care, and push back when their symptoms are dismissed. They don't have to white-knuckle their way through it.

Talk about HRT. Talk about supplements. Talk about mental health. Talk about pelvic floor therapy. Normalize the conversation so they know what to expect and so they feel prepared to advocate for themselves when the time comes.

Your Story = Their Roadmap

Every time you speak openly about menopause, you make it easier for someone else to do the same. Every time you share a piece of wisdom, you empower someone else to navigate this transition with more confidence and clarity.

When the next generation faces menopause, they'll remember what you told them. They'll remember that it's messy, unpredictable, and sometimes completely unhinged—but also transformative and powerful. They'll know they can handle it because you showed them how.

You survived it. You thrived through it. Now you're handing down the blueprint so they can thrive too.

Thriving Through Personal Growth and Transformation

KEY Takeaways

1. Menopause marks a powerful rebirth, not a decline.
2. Small steps build lasting resilience and momentum.
3. Sharing your truth helps others find theirs.

HOT TIPs

- ◆ Create your own definition of success for this season.
- ◆ Celebrate what you've survived—then dream bigger.
- ◆ Bold reinvention often starts with "Why the hell not?"

ACTION ITEMS

- ☐ Write a letter to your future self five years from now.
- ☐ Create a "hell yes" vision board.
- ☐ Pick one goal and map 3 small steps to move toward it.
- ☐ Support or mentor one woman just entering menopause.

✦ Resources ✦

- Website: getguru.com — SMART Goals templates
- Book: Menopausing by Davina McCall and Dr. Naomi Potter
- Instagram: @tamsenfadal
- Podcast: The Next Chapter Experience with Janette Blissett

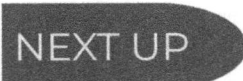 *The conclusion is your rally cry. You're not just surviving—you're thriving, leading, and redefining midlife on your own terms.*

CONCLUSION

As we reach the end of our journey together, I want to reflect on the incredible path we've traveled. Throughout this book, we've explored the transformative power of menopause, diving deep into the physical, emotional, and social aspects of this life-changing phase. We've tackled the challenges head-on, from managing hot flashes and mood swings to navigating relationships and redefining our sense of self. Together, we've discovered that menopause is not an ending, but a beginning—a catalyst for personal growth, empowerment, and reinvention.

Looking back, we've covered so much ground. We've learned effective strategies for managing symptoms, like incorporating lifestyle changes, exploring natural remedies, and working with healthcare professionals to find the right treatment plan. We've delved into the emotional landscape of menopause, discussing the importance of self-care, stress management, and building a supportive network. We've also explored the social and cultural aspects of menopause, breaking down stigmas and encouraging open, honest conversations about this natural phase of life.

But more than just a collection of information and strategies, this book has been a journey of empowerment. By understanding the science behind menopause, sharing our stories, and embracing the changes we face, we've discovered a newfound strength and resilience. We've learned that menopause is not something to be feared or ashamed of, but an opportunity to thrive and embrace our authentic selves.

As you reflect on your own menopause journey, I encourage you to consider how you can apply the insights and strategies from this book to your personal life. Whether it's trying a new exercise routine, exploring mindfulness practices, or reaching out to friends and family for support, every small step can make a big difference. Remember, menopause is a unique experience for every woman, and there's no one-size-fits-all approach. Trust your instincts, listen to your body, and don't be afraid to advocate for your needs.

But the journey doesn't end here. Please take the knowledge and empowerment you've gained and pay it forward. Join or form a support group, share your experiences with others, and help break down the stigma surrounding menopause. By engaging in open, honest conversations, we can create a sense of community and belonging, reminding each other that we're not alone on this path.

As you move forward, keep setting goals and exploring new passions. Menopause is just the beginning of a new chapter, filled with opportunities for personal growth and reinvention. Embrace the changes, celebrate your strengths, and never stop learning and growing. Whether it's taking up a new hobby, traveling to new places, or pursuing a long-held dream, this is your time to thrive.

Before we part ways, I want to express my deepest gratitude for joining me on this journey. Your courage, openness, and willingness to embrace change inspire me every day. As a lifelong advocate for believing in yourself and tackling life head-on, I know that you have the strength and resilience to navigate this phase with grace and determination. Remember, you are not alone, and by embracing your unique path, you can create a life that is truly extraordinary.

So here's to you, my fellow menopause warrior. May you continue to thrive, grow, and embrace the incredible woman you are. Keep shining bright, supporting others, and never forget the power that lies within you. The best is yet to come.

With love and gratitude,

Kim "Rocket Mean" Stegeman

REFERENCES

- American Psychological Association. (2019). Mindfulness meditation: A research-proven way to reduce stress. https://www.apa.org/topics/mindfulness/meditation
- Balance Menopause. (2021). Menopause and relationships: A guide for partners. Retrieved from https://balance-menopause.com/uploads/2021/09/Menopause-and-relationships-Feb-22.pdf
- BSW Health. (n.d.). Women's wellness: How to be your best self in your 40s. Retrieved from https://www.bswhealth.com/blog/women-health-forties
- Burn Fat and Feast. (n.d.). Mindful eating for menopausal women. Retrieved from https://burnfatandfeast.com/mindful-eating-for-menopausal-women/
- Canada Coach Academy. (n.d.). Become a menopause coach in 2025: The complete guide. Retrieved from https://canadacoachacademy.com/become-a-menopause-coach/#:~:text=A%20menopause%20coach%20is%20a,changes%20of%20this%20life%20stage
- Celebrities who have spoken out about menopause. (n.d.). Glamour. Retrieved from https://www.glamour.com/gallery/celebrities-who-have-spoken-out-about-menopause
- Cramer, H., Lauche, R., & Dobos, G. (2019). Mindfulness-based stress reduction for menopausal symptoms after risk-reducing salpingo-oophorectomy: A randomized controlled trial. BJOG: An International Journal of Obstetrics & Gynaecology, 126(8), 1036–1044. https://doi.org/10.1111/1471-0528.15471
- Dewa, C. S., Loong, D., Bonato, S., & Joosen, M. C. W. (2023). Effectiveness of stress management interventions to change cortisol in health professionals: A meta-analysis. Psychoneuroendocrinology, 153, 105229. https://doi.org/10.1016/j.psyneuen.2023.105229
- FemmePharma. (n.d.). Understanding Medicare coverage for menopause-related healthcare. Retrieved from https://femmepharma.com/understanding-medicare-coverage-for-menopause-related-healthcare/
- Gennev. (2021). Menopause and exercise: Endorphin boosters. Retrieved from https://www.gennev.com/learn/menopause-and-exercise
- Gennev. (n.d.). How to counteract stress in menopause: Resiliency.

- Retrieved from https://www.gennev.com/learn/stress-menopause-resiliency
- Gunter, J. (2021). The menopause manifesto: Own your health with facts and feminism. Kensington Books.
- Guru. (n.d.). How to write SMART goals: With examples. Retrieved from https://www.getguru.com/reference/smart-goals
- Harvard Health Publishing. (n.d.). Menopause and mental health. Retrieved from https://www.health.harvard.edu/womens-health/menopause-and-mental-health
- Health.com. (2025). Exercise to manage menopause weight gain and other symptoms. Retrieved from https://www.health.com/menopause-exercise-8784762
- Healthline. (n.d.). 12 science-based benefits of meditation. Retrieved from https://www.healthline.com/nutrition/12-benefits-of-meditation
- Healthline. (n.d.). Menopause diet: How what you eat affects your symptoms. Retrieved from https://www.healthline.com/nutrition/menopause-diet
- Healthline. (n.d.). Menopause: Tips for talking to your doctor. Retrieved from https://www.healthline.com/health/menopause/talking-with-your-doctor#:~:text=That's%20why%20it's%20so%20important,to%20help%20manage%20your%20symptoms
- HealthyWomen. (n.d.). You're hot. Vasomotor symptoms are not. Retrieved from https://www.healthywomen.org/your-health/cooling-products-for-vasomotor-symptoms
- Johns Hopkins Medicine. (n.d.). Can menopause cause depression? Retrieved from https://www.hopkinsmedicine.org/health/wellness-and-prevention/can-menopause-cause-depression#:~:text=Hormonal%20Fluctuations&text=When%20hormone%20levels%20drop,%20serotonin,let%20roll%20off%20your%20back
- Johns Hopkins Medicine. (n.d.). Introduction to menopause. Retrieved from https://www.hopkinsmedicine.org/health/conditions-and-diseases/introduction-to-menopause
- Khajehei, M., Rajaei, S., & Aghaz, A. (2021). Effect of mindfulness-based counseling on sexual self-efficacy and sexual satisfaction among Iranian postmenopausal women. The Journal of Sexual Medicine, 18(8), 1338–1345. https://www.ncbi.nlm.nih.gov/pmc/articles/PMC10318424/
- Mayo Clinic Press. (n.d.). Menopause facts vs. fiction: The truth behind the myths. Retrieved from https://mcpress.mayoclinic.org/menopause/common-myths-of-menopause/

- Mayo Clinic. (n.d.). Bioidentical hormones: Are they safer? Retrieved from https://www.mayoclinic.org/diseases-conditions/menopause/expert-answers/bioidentical-hormones/faq-20058460
- McCall, D., & Potter, N. (2022). Menopausing: The positive roadmap to your second spring. HarperCollins.
- Menopause Journal. (2024). Effects of mind-body exercise on perimenopausal and menopausal symptoms. Retrieved from https://journals.lww.com/menopausejournal/fulltext/2024/05000/effects_of_mind_body_exercise_on_perimenopausal.13.aspx
- Mindful.org. (n.d.). Navigating menopause: A mindful approach to managing symptoms and embracing change. Retrieved from https://www.mindful.org/navigating-menopause-a-mindful-approach-to-managing-symptoms-and-embracing-change/
- My Menoplan. (n.d.). Women's stories. Retrieved from https://mymenoplan.org/womens-stories/
- Naomi Watts candidly discusses early menopause. (n.d.). InStyle. Retrieved from https://www.instyle.com/naomi-watts-never-work-again-menopause-8773169
- National Center for Biotechnology Information. (n.d.). Acupuncture in menopause (AIM) study. Retrieved from https://pmc.ncbi.nlm.nih.gov/articles/PMC4874921/#:~:text=A%20recent%20meta%2Danalysis%20of,lasting%20up%20to%203%20months
- National Center for Biotechnology Information. (n.d.). Exercise beyond menopause: Dos and don'ts. Retrieved from https://pmc.ncbi.nlm.nih.gov/articles/PMC3296386/
- National Center for Biotechnology Information. (n.d.). Herbal products used in menopause. Retrieved from https://pmc.ncbi.nlm.nih.gov/articles/PMC8708702/
- National Menopause Foundation. (n.d.). Community. Retrieved from https://nationalmenopausefoundation.org/community/
- Neff, K. D. (n.d.). Self-compassion: What is self-compassion? Retrieved from https://self-compassion.org/what-is-self-compassion/
- NHS Inform. (n.d.). Menopause and your mental wellbeing. Retrieved from https://www.nhsinform.scot/healthy-living/womens-health/later-years-around-50-years-and-over/menopause-and-post-menopause-health/menopause-and-your-mental-wellbeing/
- NHS Inform. (n.d.). Supporting someone through menopause. Retrieved from https://www.nhsinform.scot/healthy-living/womens-health/later-years-around-50-years-and-over/menopause-and-post-menopause-health/supporting-someone-through-the-menopause/#:~:text=Communication%20is%20key
- North American Menopause Society. (n.d.). Choosing a healthcare

- practitioner. Retrieved from https://menopause.org/patient-education/choosing-a-healthcare-practitioner
- Northrup, C. (2012). The wisdom of menopause: Creating physical and emotional health during the change (3rd ed.). Bantam Books.
- Office on Women's Health. (n.d.). Menopause and sexuality. Retrieved from https://womenshealth.gov/menopause/menopause-and-sexuality
- Phaptuech, Y., Sitthimongkol, Y., & Wiroteurairuang, T. (2013). Effects of mindfulness meditation on serum cortisol of medical students. Journal of the Medical Association of Thailand, 96(Suppl 1), S90–S95. https://pubmed.ncbi.nlm.nih.gov/23724462/
- Purely Calm. (n.d.). 40 amazing hobbies for women in their 40s. Retrieved from https://www.purelycalm.com/40-hobbies-for-women-in-their-40s/
- Rupa Health. (2024). Cortisol & its impact on menopause (with tips to manage cortisol). Retrieved from https://www.rupahealth.com/post/cortisol-and-menopause
- StatPearls. (n.d.). Hormone replacement therapy. Retrieved from https://www.ncbi.nlm.nih.gov/books/NBK493191/
- StatPearls. (n.d.). Menopause. Retrieved from https://www.ncbi.nlm.nih.gov/books/NBK507826/
- University of Utah Health. (2019). How to practice self-compassion for resilience and well-being. Retrieved from https://accelerate.uofuhealth.utah.edu/resilience/how-to-practice-self-compassion-for-resilience-and-well-being
- UR Medicine. (2025). Self-compassion and your mental health. Retrieved from https://www.urmc.rochester.edu/behavioral-health-partners/bhp-blog/february-2025/self-compassion-and-your-mental-health
- Verywell Health. (2024). 12 benefits of regular exercise, backed by research. Retrieved from https://www.verywellhealth.com/benefits-of-exercise-8704494
- WebMD. (n.d.). Natural treatments for menopause symptoms. Retrieved from https://www.webmd.com/menopause/menopause-natural-treatments
- Özcan, A. G., & Yılmaz, E. (2021). The effect of breathing exercise on stress hormones. Cyprus Journal of Medical Sciences, 6(2), 107–112. https://doi.org/10.5152/cjms.2021.2020.2390

www.ingramcontent.com/pod-product-compliance
Lightning Source LLC
Chambersburg PA
CBHW020457030426
42337CB00011B/141